# YOUR HOMEMADE NATURAL PRODUCTS

*THE COMPLETE GUIDE TO DO-IT-YOURSELF BODY CARE, BUTTERS, BATH, LOTIONS AND ORGANIC RECIPES*

© Copyright 2020 by ProWellness Publishing
All rights reserved.

This document is geared towards providing exact and reliable information with regards to the topic and issue covered. The publication is sold with the idea that the publisher is not required to render accounting, officially permitted, or otherwise, qualified services. If advice is necessary, legal or professional, a practiced individual in the profession should be ordered.

- From a Declaration of Principles which was accepted and approved equally by a Committee of the American Bar Association and a Committee of Publishers and Associations.

In no way is it legal to reproduce, duplicate, or transmit any part of this document in either electronic means or in printed format. Recording of this publication is strictly prohibited and any storage of this document is not allowed unless with written permission from the publisher. All rights reserved.

The information provided herein is stated to be truthful and consistent, in that any liability, in terms of inattention or otherwise, by any usage or abuse of any policies, processes, or directions contained within is the solitary and utter responsibility of the recipient reader. Under no circumstances will any legal responsibility or blame be held against the publisher for any reparation, damages, or monetary loss due to the information herein, either directly or indirectly.

Respective authors own all copyrights not held by the publisher.

The information herein is offered for informational purposes solely, and is universal as so. The presentation of the information is without contract or any type of guarantee assurance.
The trademarks that are used are without any consent, and the publication of the trademark is without permission or backing by the trademark owner. All trademarks and brands within this book are for clarifying purposes only and are the owned by the owners themselves, not affiliated with this document.

Page left intentionally blank

Table of Contents

Somebody has a query about the best ways to experience ingredients just beginning with their own homemade cleaning supplies, especially when looking for specialty ingredients such as essential oils. Thankfully, it's easy to create homemade cleaners, with a lot of supplies available in your local foodstuffs or discount shop.

It is simple, inexpensive, and fun to make homemade cleaning products. One of the best things about natural cleaners is that they are often made from the same simple ingredients. Here are a few things to do with your recipes if you start making your own natural cleaning products.

People put a lot of confidence in the efficacy of the treatments for homemade natural skincare, but the question is that they are the same as other sources claim. Magazines and websites always offer recipes for different mixtures that they say do wonder for your skin, and people like the idea that their anti-aging products will cost them almost no money.

Creating your own spa, as well as skincare products, can or cannot resolve several small problems in your skin. It depends only on personal preference and maybe some common sense. You will know what to do while dealing with foods and how to find relief from skin pain, but please try to receive medical treatment first to make sure it is appropriately handled.

# IMPORTANCE OF 100% NATURAL PRODUCTS (NATURAL PRODUCTS BENEFIT)

## Homemade Natural Beauty Products

Homemade natural beauty products enable you to enjoy the comfort of your home. You will feel happy to learn that you use more natural goods that are much safer for you than heavily manufactured shop labels.

Facial mask revitalization

As the skin ages, this could appear exhausted and gray. Having frequent facial medication helps to reduce the signs of aging and reverses stress, ultraviolet ray exposure, and even acne skin damage. Using the following for a mask that not only lightens the skin but also exfoliates:

- 1 tomato overripe
- 1 teaspoon citrus fruit juice
- 1 teaspoon oatmeal instantly

Puree all ingredients in a blender before they are mixed. Kindly adhere to the face and remove it before rinsing with warm water for 30 minutes.

Facial Powder Hydrating

Hydrated skin is good skin. With this night cream recipe, keeping your skin hydrated is simple. The following are needed:

- 3 lanolin cubits.
- 1 charcoal sunflower oil.
- 1 charcoal almond oi;
- 1 tea Kuchar wash oil.

Melt the lanolin with a double boiler. Attach the sunflower and almond oil when soft, blend well. Clear from the sun and relax for a moment. As the mixture becomes thick, add the lavender oil. Place the mixture in a jar that is airtight.

Face Balm Tinted

For handmade items of natural beauty that give a touch of color to the lips and also have the following shiny shine:

10 Fresh Cranberries-You can use more berries before you have the darkness or for a brighter hue, the amount of berries you use before you have exceeded the ideal lightness.

- 1 charcoal of almond oil
- 1 tablespoon sweetheart
- 1 Vitamin E oil decline

Place all ingredients in a healthy bowl with a microwave. Two minutes of the fast microwave, or before the mixture begins to boil. This can also be achieved if desired on top of the pot. Mix well and break pulp berries. Allow the mixture to cool; remove the cranberry pulp with a strainer. Stir again before switching to a plastic tub.

Skin scrub exfoliating

Good, silky skin in season, irrespective of the time of year. Household natural beauty products such as this exfoliating body scrub can be easily created using the following ingredients:

- 2 1/2 cups of source.
- 1/2 cup of almond sweet oil
- 4 tea cubes citrus concentrate.
- 4 tablespoons of sweetheart
- Four drops of essential lemon oil

In a large bowl, combine the sugar and the sweet almond oil, mixing well. Add the citrus juice before adding essential lemon oil and honey. Remove the mixture until all components are spread equally.

Calming lotion of body

Use the following for an aromatic body lotion suitable for stress-relief:

- 1 charcoal lanolin.
- 2 tea cubes of sugar.
- 2 tea cubes of chamomile oil.

• 2 tea cubes of washing oil.

Melt the lanolin with chamomile and lavender oil with a double boiler. Until pouring into a sealable container, extract from heat, and cool. Following exfoliation, massage a lotion in the skin to keep the skin moisturized.

Homemade natural beauty products were also simple and eco-friendly products that you can make at home. You control the quality of the ingredients and can change each recipe according to your liking and dislike.

### All-Natural Products - Should We Use Them?

Practical or unpractical?

Today, the environment is a hot topic. You see and hear the word 'green' on TV, radio, and news, and it's everywhere. If you actually stop thinking, it is meaningful to use all-natural products. Why not, if it is good for us and the environment, I 'd use it. But the main question is whether it's practical or not.

When you shop, what are the most critical aspects of your decision to purchases? Two things come to mind: time and costs. Firstly, which store is the most convenient for the product you want. Secondly, the best price based on quality is one of the product choices.

The answer is obvious; the most products we have at our convenience are not all-natural or earth-friendly. In addition, if All-natural products are available, the cost can be higher. However, the availability of these products has greatly improved, and the internet provides a convenient way for us to shop.

What's the advantage?

Health and environment.
It's pretty easy to understand why one has an effect on the other. When we eat organic products, free of toxins and contaminants, we are growing the poisons we consume so that we have a better diet.
If we choose earth-friendly products and lower our demand for products that harm our environment, we will gradually reduce pollutants in the air, soil, and water. Thus, as our conditions improve on the environment, it follows that our health will benefit as well.

To sum up:
Today, while it can't be entirely feasible to use all-natural goods, with a growing understanding of the public contributing to higher competition, we can see more variety at a reduced cost. In fact, the rise of internet shopping can make such items more accessible for purchases.

Amazing Aloe Vera Products Benefits for Your Skin

The advantages of products Aloe Vera cannot be ignored.

Health and soothing qualities are two of the attributes of Aloe Vera goods known to people for decades. Although there are several types of pills and alternatives available in the contemporary world today to cure the diseases, people are dependent and reliable on natural cure techniques and methods. The herb is generally popular for a variety of diseases due to the natural remedy. Thanks to its easy usability and the benefits it is gaining worldwide fame.

The product is extremely useful.

The benefit of Aloe Vera can be derived from the concentrated shape, which combines the goodness and medicinal properties of the juice with the mild citrus taste to ensure a healthy digestive system. This also has the ability to clear away the excess toxins from the body and to fix any issues pertaining to the stomach. Would you not agree that this herbal remedy is a human race boon?

The success of cosmetics

The advantages of the Aloe Vera products can also be seen by the popularity of its natural cosmetics, which people all over the world admire. These cosmetic products have gained enormous importance and attention because they contain herbal and 100 % natural elements which are deemed beneficial for healthy and soft skin maintenance. You will add shine to the face to remove all sorts of skin issues without inducing pain and feeling of burning.

The gel is a magic product.

The goods from Aloe Vera are well known and popular as they are able to fix many health issues instantly. The gel type is known as an excellent drug that can heal and soothe the eyes, burns, and other skin irritation. It is also useful for the removal of scars, defects, and anti-aging properties. The drug has positive effects on different forms of health conditions because of its antiseptic properties.

It's safe to drink raw and herbal tea.

If you want to enjoy herbal tea with natural ingredients and artificial fillers without any preservatives, you can benefit from the Aloe Vera products. It helps not only to keep your mind young and comfortable, but it also purifies your stomach and lets you keep your body clean. There are millions of people who stay healthy by drinking herbal tea. Why don't you do that too to feel the difference in your life?

Choosing the right element is crucial.
Whether in the form of gel, lotion, or as soap, oil, tea, shampoo, or other therapeutic products, those other natural items seem to be extremely effective and helpful to the human body. But when you pick up goods from so many different brands on the market, it is crucial that you make the correct decision at fair and pocket-friendly prices.

Although almost everyone agrees the use of beauty and skincare products is critical in both looking and feeling healthy, some people purchase these products simply on the basis of the success of the brand name or because some friends have shown that these products are effective.

Some people are, however, a little more cautious and careful about what chemicals they use in different parts of their bodies. These people tend to look more closely at the labels to find out the primary ingredients, be they natural or synthetic.

We always want to use the best products available when it comes to taking care of our appearance. We also want them to contain as much as possible soft but effective natural ingredients. Herbs, spices, fruits, and flowers are only a handful of the most common natural ingredients commonly used in cosmetics.

However, some may favor handmade makeup items consisting of natural ingredients similar to those sold in the supermarkets. Not only are homemade beauty products cheap, but they also have lots of other advantages over oversold cosmetic products.

Benefits

The biggest benefit of buying homemade makeup products is that you know precisely what ingredients are being used to keep you from thinking about difficult additives or toxic substances of which you are allergic.

Moreover, you should get more imaginative and add whatever natural ingredient you know to clean the face or body would make your solution more powerful.

Another big benefit of making your own natural makeup goods is that you will save a lot of time. That is because the products themselves are what you have to offer. There is no reason to think about depreciation charges and distributor discount fees.

Recipes Review

A foot scrub is one of the most popular examples of handmade beauty items, perfect for soothing sore and stressed feet. You need the following ingredients for your own foot scrub at home: a table-top of gross sand, clean sand, a cup of liquid hand soap, Epsom, salt, and canola oil. Combine both of them to make a gritty paste and rub it on foot.

A hair rinse is another easy-to-make homemade drug to apply to the makeup and skincare regimen. This is ideal for eliminating hair buildup. To make the hair better, add a teaspoon of honey and four cups of warm water. To add fragrance to your hair rinse formula, you can add a drop of your favorite sweet oil. Thoroughly apply it to your hair and scalp and let it dry.

Homemade Bath Products...the Pros and Cons

You can find other websites selling homemade bathing recipe while browsing the internet: "Why to spend extra for pricey bath goods if you are willing to produce your own stuff ... Forget (give up) these pricey bath products in bathrooms (drug, store, etc.), and you should produce your own, inexpensive bath products at home ... etc.

Is it correct? Yes and no ... Yes and no.

Let us characterize three main natural bath product levels depending on various factors. The level of sophistication of form, structure, equipment, medicinal benefit and effects, the biological function of ingredients, etc., varies from other stages.

-- Natural bath product levels: NEVER REGULAR mineral salts unscented or scented, colored or colored, etc. E.g., Epsom salt, Dead sea salts, groundwater, sea salt, salt-lake, and so on.

Can you at home make these bath salts? Yes, you could indeed ... You can ... It's easy ...

In a wash, apply the combination of bath salts, essential oils, and food colors. That's it! That's it! The recommendation "make at home" for this type of bath items is also the best and best recommendation. You can produce this type of inexpensive bath items at home.

Homemade possibility: Yes, in your home spa, it is easy to make this kind of product.

Pros: Simple and cheap bath products. Pros:

Conditions: This basic arrangement reduces medical ability and advantages. The results depend directly on the quantity of products added to the water. The more ..., the more you add.

-- Natural bath products level MIDDLE: MUD baths (organic, mineral), HERBAL baths with plain, herbal oils, aroma oils, and milk baths, etc.

The structure and medicinal benefit of this class of bath products are more nuanced. This class needs more energy, more commitment, and more information at home.

You obviously can't make regular mud baths. Instead, you buy a ready mud extract – Dead Sea Mud, Moor Mud, etc.

Even other bath products can be made at home (milk baths, herbal baths).

To boil tea, add dried herbs, steam, sprinkle with sugar, blend with salts or condensed milk, apply essential oils.

Homemade possibility: Yes, for some products, it is possible (but not simple).

Pros: Active additives give home spa baths more medicinal and health benefits.

Contrary: More time, effort, and knowledge are required for this class. Unfortunately, so several therapeutic ingredients of such a class cannot penetrate the skin when they are prepared and produced at home. This reduces the therapeutic value.

-- Advance natural bath products levels: creative, holistic bath products with new principles, inventions, design, and holistic expertise with SMART properties and behavior. These products provide a full range of both experience and value, together with the benefits of major bath products.

This kind of natural bath items could not be made at home. Complex ingredients scientific steps, Special technology, innovations, new ideas, clinical studies, exclusive solutions. e.tc., are required to demonstrate advanced value.

This class is intended for advanced bathers who are trying to experience more interesting ideas as well as products than regular products on the mass market.

Homemade: Sorry, at home you can't do this lesson.

Pros: More nuanced structure provides intellectual control of more medicinal benefits, ranges, good outcomes. Biological behavior and intelligent interest are now the primary therapeutic center. The intelligent ... the better.

Opposite: This class is not easy to find. Such products are also only sold on specialist treatment markets (water massage, hydrotherapy).

Do you need this class samples? Please don't let the producers know this notion!

Idea: Try to combine main bath products in one bathroom at home:

- Salts of Bath
- Bath of mud
- Herbal bathing
- Bath of Thalassa
- Bath of flavor

It is not an easy and simple task ... I'd predict it's going to be a nightmare to combine them into one Bath.

### *Do Homemade Natural Skin Care Recipes Actually Work?*

People have a great deal of confidence in the efficacy of their own natural skincare remedy, but the question is, are these combinations as many sources claim. Magazines and web pages also sell recipes for various mixtures, which they believe would do wonders for the skin, and consumers like the fact that their anti-aging products would practically cost them absolutely nothing. You get what you're asking for sometimes.

People turn to these formulas not just because they save money but also because they are frustrated by the counter-skin care formulas they have used. The cosmetics companies usually supply products that do not fulfill their promises of efficiency and frequently contain a lot of unpleasant ingredients. Many of the chemicals in these products will potentially hurt you, and you have to be careful about what you buy.

Homemade natural skincare formulations are certainly better than the norm, as the packaged goods are usually packed with chemicals. These do not give you more incentives than the formulations purchased in the supermarket. When using these ingredients, what you really want to give your skin is antioxidants and a few basic nutrients.

Not that I say that it is not extremely useful to provide the skin with vitamins, minerals, and essential fatty acids, and antioxidants are an absolute must for good health. Antioxidants can make you appear younger by avoiding the harm done by free radicals that snatch electrons from the skin that are part of a chemical system. What I mean is more needs to be done if you want to make your skin firmer and smoother.

You lose collagen, elastin, and hyaluronic acid at an increasing pace because these compounds break down because of the action of the enzymes. Your levels of collagen and elastin production have also collapsed, and your homemade natural skincare is nearly impossible. Avocado oil can be used to promote collagen production, but you need components that are stronger than this material alone.

The only way to combat all-natural anti-aging skin care products is to address tissue and polymer degradation and manufacturing difficulties. This is achieved by mixing Phytessence Wakame Help, grape seed oil, and Cinergy TK and Nano-Lipoble H EQ10 compounds. The two last molecules, however, come from protein complexes, enzymes, and a nano-emulsified form of Q10 coenzyme.

Phytessence Phytessence Wakame and grape seed oil help you preserve the collagen, elastin, and hyaluronic acid supply by control of the degradation of the enzymes. Cynergy TK and Nano-Lipobelle build tissue supply by dramatically increasing your production of collagen and elastin. The result such ingredients can achieve cannot be accomplished by a homemade natural skincare recipe.

By using items that contain the right mix of ingredients, you will do better than homemade natural skincare.

Natural Products for Your Baby's Skin

Practical or unpractical?

The environment is currently a hot topic. You're watching and listening to the 'Green' word on TV, radio, and news, everywhere. When you finally avoid worrying about it, it makes sense to use all-natural ingredients. Why not, because it benefits people and the community, I can definitely do it. But the main issue is whether it's realistic or not.

What are the most significant factors in your purchasing decision when you shop? There are two things to remember; time and expense. First, which shop is the most convenient to supply your desired products. Secondly, among the commodity options, which one has the best quality rates.

The answer is obvious: most of our products are not all-natural or land friendly in a convenient place. In fact, the cost will be higher where all-natural goods are available. The range of these items has, therefore, vastly increased, and the internet provides an easy place to buy. As competition increases, we should all expect more natural options at a lower rate.

What's the advantage?

Health and environment.

It's very easy to see that one has an effect on the other. If we prefer organic, pesticide-free, and chemical fertilizers, we that the toxins we consume and have healthy food for ourselves. This helps our bodies to battle death more quickly.

If we choose earth-friendly products and reduce our demand for products that harm our environment, we will gradually reduce pollutants in the air, on the ground, and in the water. Thus, as our environmental situations change, our health will also benefit.

To sum up:

Today, it may not be fully feasible to use all-natural goods, but we will see larger variations at a lower price with an increased market perception that adds to growing competition. In addition, these products will become more convenient to buy with the growth of internet shopping. When we purchase and consume goods that are not toxic to us and the world, a healthier environment can help both our families and future generations.

## All-Natural Indulgences

Do you know that your own cosmetic products, spa treatments, and organic beauty products can be made? Not just this would save you a lot of money by making your own goods and keep you from placing dangerous substances on your bodies. We only think of eating, drinking, or breathing chemicals; nevertheless, the skin is an organ, and chemicals placed on our skin are absorbed and enter our blood and move to all our organs. Do you understand why the chemicals in commercially formulated skincare products are so important to avoid?

You can create homemade skincare products that are cheaper, easier, and safer than store-bought versions. We can avoid allergic reactions to the harsh chemicals of commercial products with precisely what goes on in our own homemade beauty products. Why not make your own skincare goods, if you consider creams or lotions that don't contain irritating fragrances hard? In this way, you can add scents that are appropriate to you or opt not to add any. In making natural beauty goods, we will also prevent nasty preservatives that cover after a beauty product has long ago been used.

The good thing is that you will enjoy natural DIY makeup products without toxic penny additives in your own house. The possibilities that you can make homemade beauty goods are almost infinite. You will make skin scrubs, lotions, face creams and body butter, lip hoops, glosses, and more. Just at home, you should make your own soaps and shampoos. Don't forget that you can even make your own natural spa items quickly and conveniently, for example, bath salts, oils, and soaks. If you usually spend a lot of money to wax your legs every month, with just sugar, water, and lemon juice, you can make an easy wax substitute.

It can be fun and gratifying to mix with your own natural homemade beauty goods. For example, if you want to experiment and make wonderful soaps as you see in many specialty shops, the method of melting and pouring soap is really quite easy. Just melt a glycerin-based soap, which is easily found in many hobby stores or online, then add the choice of essential fragrance oils, finally add your soap color and mold. You may also apply glitter or furnishings to your wash, such as little seashells. It's so easy that older kids can do it with little guidance.

## Homemade Beauty Recipes

The cosmetics company has been a multi-million - dollar market over the decades. Not one year passes without the introduction of a new cosmetic or beauty scheme. While all of these cosmetic remedies, while exciting, can be, others would also do more harm to the skin or hair for a long time. It is, therefore, not surprising that women look for homemade natural alternatives to the chemical compound treatments they have used until now.

Here are some wonderful homemade beauty recipes you definitely have to try ...

Homemade makeup face recipe: banana and strawberry mask

The trick to rectify this is by using a moisturizing mask made of banana and honey if your skin is dry and flaccid. A ripe banana curries. Add two or three teaspoons of sweetheart. Combine the blend very well. Apply the mixture cautiously to coat the whole face and back. Let it linger 10 to 15 minutes on your forehead. Flush it all with clean water.

Homemade blackhead beauty recipe: Papaya as well as milk exfoliation mask

Nose and chin blackheads more often than not require medical treatment, which can be very painful. However, with a soft exfoliation mask made from papaya and milk, you can quickly clear blackheads without discomfort. Mash half mature papaya with two teaspoons of milk. Apply the paste to the face and massage it with your fingers softly onto the eyes. The Papaya enzyme hastens the pores of your skin to unclog and speeds up the removal of dead skin cells and dirt.

Homemade Makeup Recipe: Horseradish with Vinegar Mask for Dark Spots

Colored or black stains may be very nonsensical on the skin. Sadly, many of the cosmetics which can remove these spots on the skin are very severe. Because of using these removers, a radish and a vinegar mask can be combined that still works well. Grate the horseradish as well as squeeze the whole juice out. Add a few drops of apple cider vinegar to the horseradish juice. In the mixture, tear a cotton ball and apply it to your dark spots. Let it linger 15-20 minutes on your face and then rinse off. With better results, add the mixture 2-3 days a week.

Homemade makeup formula for eye bluffness and dark circles: cucumber and potato mask

One of the worst facial issues to contend with is dark circles under the lips. Eyelids can also get puffy in some situations. A potato and a cucumber mask were the perfect treatment. Grate and add with the whole potato and the cucumber. Apply the mixture to the eyes closed and require 10-15 minutes to live. When time is up, clean your hair.

Casual skin Hands Recipe: Lemon and Sugar Scrub

While we tend to concentrate more often on the face, we tend to forget that our hands must also be beautiful. It may be disconcerting to have a pretty face, but because of your everyday work, your hands are rough and dirty and wrinkled. One way to keep your hands clean, gentle, and clear is to use an exfoliator made up of natural ingredients such as citrus and sugar. In a small pot, place 2-3 tablespoons of granulated sugar and squash either lemons or lime juice. Mix it up, but make sure that the sugar is not fully absorbed in the water. Massage the skin softly until the granules of sugar fully dissolve. In cold water, clean your mouth.

Know more homemade recipe for beauty





Let's be frank, what else does all the leftover pumpkin you have from Halloween have to do? Buckets and buckets of the things you did with them, all of the insides of those carving jobs. There's just so much pumpkin pastry that you can make, and it's not a recipe for everyone. There's something you can do about it, but ...

Pumpkin DIY Recipes for Beauty

You have a very intelligent way to save a little Christmas fortune here if you play your cards correctly. The pumpkin season is here, and this is great because both eating pumpkin and plastering them all over your face offers so many benefits. However, come Christmas, there are fewer calves so that you cannot reap the advantages that nutrient-rich food has to offer.

Provide your friends and family with these pumpkin DIY makeup tips all year long. Place them in vintage, reusable bottles, wrap around them a festive ribbon, and what do you have? A bunch of presents ready for Christmas. And happy to stay available if a missed friend keeps staying ...

The good thing is the pumpkin can be frozen too! The raw meat should be sliced into chunks and put into freezer bags. You might also purify the meat and pack it into ice cube traps if you like. For a fast substitute, if you need a mask at the last minute, this is a perfect idea. Plus, you 're going to have some realistic for the spice lattes you like when coffee shops stop making them ...

There are so many makeup items you can make from Halloween from all the leftover pumpkin. So long as you follow the instructions right and stock the items accordingly, you have your very own unique collection of cosmetics and therapies, which in turn offer far more advantages than the expensive shops you have bought.


Spiced Pumpkin Sugar Scrub Squares

For Christmas, this is such a perfect idea, plus you can use those holiday ice cube trays you never want to use too! Using them as molds to make pumpkin spiced sugar scrub shapes and squares ideally suited for a Christmassy pumpkin DIY beauty recipe in an old pot.

A quarter a cup of coconut oil, a cup of brown sugar, half a cup of scentless, powdered soap, a teaspoon of pure pumpkin, and a teaspoon of pumpkin spice or cinnamon are only desired.

This recipe can be changed according to your own tastes, and you may also add coffee beans, maple syrup, white sugar, or anything you want to blend. It's all about trial and error, so try it and have some fun.

The sugar in this recipe serves as a natural exfoliant for the skin, so if you blend with antioxidants so enzymes in the pumpkin 's flesh, you have plenty that can effectively fight wrinkles and produce a vibrant face. The old skin cells are rubbed off with raw sugar. The chocolate oil helps to complete it with a perfect, dense, comfortable body moisturizer to make you feel smooth for days.

Fix-It Mask Pumpkin & Honey

You'll probably find your face the first place that gives you the game if you've been partying hard or just working for too many hours. Your skin can be gray and sallow, and wrinkles or dark circles more apparent than they used to be. You can get all these stuffs out in just as soon as you sit with the pumpkin and delicious face mask – yet another of the pumpkin DIY beauty recipes, you can put into a bowl and give for Christmas to a family or a friend!

If you'd like to make a single face mask, you need it:

Cinnamon 1/2 tsp

1/2 tsp of dairy

1/2 tsp sweetheart

Purified pumpkin 2 tsp

This is more of a kind of recipe that you need as milk becomes a treatment that will not last even longer than a week when stored in the refrigerator. If you are ready to use, mix it together, add your face, sit and relax 10 minutes before you wash off.

The honey throughout this recipe is a humectant that keeps moisture. This helps preserve the moisture on the face while pumpkin-flesh antioxidants magically supply the skin cells with the nutrients they need. The milk helps cool and cure all sore areas, and cinnamon-this serves as a natural cleanser, but if the skin is allergic, it can be removed. Just leave it. Just leave it.

There are so many DIY beauty pumpkin recipes that you can use with all the remaining pumpkin you have in Halloween. Neither should you dwell on these Christmas gifts-with all the advantages that this food can offer your skin, and you should easily relax. You don't need that many ingredients, and only pennies are required for treatments. There are lots of body parts you could relax after Halloween with face masks, sugar scrubs, hair enhancers, pedicure treatments, and more.

Natural Beauty Recipes - Pamper Yourself from Head to Toe Naturally

The best recipes of natural beauty are those which contain only the best natural ingredients that support your skin. The best way to ensure that your beauty products contain 100 % natural ingredients is to create them yourself so you can make several natural makeup recipes at home.

You don't have to pay high market rates to feed and soothe your skin. Yes, natural alternatives are also both safer and often more successful than the chemical-charged makeup goods on the high street for sale.

Try these basic homemade recipes for your skin, body,  hair, feet, and hands, of natural beauty:

Natural Beauty Recipes 1 — Facial Mask with Papaya Enzyme (Exfoliate and Face Nourish)

This facial mask is among the most famous recipes of natural beauty.

The following ingredients are needed:

1/2 cup of mashed papaya, 1 cup of white egg, and 1 cup of sugar. Add a tablespoon of plain yogurt to the mixture for additional cooling, as well as if you have sensitive skin.

Type:

In a large pot, combine all the ingredients together. Before applying the facial mask combination, make sure you wash your hair. Keep the mask on your face for about 5 to 8 minutes, allowing the papayas enzymes time to clean your scalp.

Then shower off with warm water, and with cooler water.

2-Herbal Vinegar Rinse for the Hair (For Gorgeous Hair)

This herbal vinegar rinse would preserve the normal pH balance in your hair, clean up dirt and hair, and reduce the olive oil in your hair.

The following ingredients are needed:

Two rosemary sprigs, two lavender sprigs, and 2 teacups. One or two tablespoons of vinegar or white vinegar.

Type:

Placed two rosemary sprigs and two lavender sprigs in 2 cups of water in such a clear glass pot. Let the container rest between 2 and 4 hours in the sun to kill the grass. Add an apple cider vinegar as well as white vinegar to the water solution with 1 or 2 tablespoons and use the same shampoo.

3-Herbal Bath Salts (Invigorate but Pamper the Body) natural beauty Recipes

Another top natural beauty recipe you could even make at home are herbal bath salts. Everything you need is a cup of sea salt and a few herbs, including rosemary, lavender, peppermint, or spearmint which are on hand.

Type:

Grind the herbs to a fine powder with a coffee grinder. Mix the salt and add a calming intensity to your next soak.

Natural Beauty Recipes 4-Flower Based Soothing Foot Soak (Refresh the Feet)

You may make different recipes of natural beauty close to this soothing flower-based foot soak.

You need sea salt for this, along with fresh-cut citrus (limes, lemons, oranges, etc.) and some flower petal selected from your garden.

Type:

Fill a small basin with lukewarm water and apply oil, petals of flowers, and slices of fruit. Soak your feet for ten minutes in a mixture, and then rinse and dry them with a soft towel.

Natural Beauty Recipes 5 – Mask of Strawberry Manicure.

This strawberry manicure mask is an excellent way to naturally spoil your hands.

Ingredients: Ingredients

3-5 ripe strawberries, a tablespoon of sugar, and the preference of light oil.

Type:

Mash 3-5 ripe strawberries, drain the juice and mix a tablespoon of sugar with a little bit of the light oil. Use a circular motion to apply the resulting mixture to your hands.

It softens and exfoliates the skin, which renders it flat, which shiny.

6-Watermelon Pedicure Paint (For Lovely Feet) Ingredients with natural beauty

This pedicure polish is perfect for your feet during the watermelon season and gives your home a pleasant aroma in the summer.

Combine 1/2 cup of mashed and strong watermelon and a teaspoon of finely ground almonds with 1/4 cup of easy yogurt.

Type:

Apply the mixture by operating in a circular pattern with your fingertips. To strip, rinse, and pat dry to enjoy the results, using a tissue.

Do not produce larger amounts than you can use. When you make more than you want, keep the excess in a refrigerator and use it in 48 hours as these organic natural beauty recipes contain no preservatives.

Natural Skin Care - More Than Skin Deep

Does Natural mean good in Skin Care?

Though Webster describes "real" as "not organic, manufactured, or naturally obtained," this is the unusual cosmetic product that fits the term. Water is also generally distilled, deionized, or otherwise purified in cosmetics. Throughout the spectrum of 'normal' goods, decisions were taken to emulsify, preserve, and retain – to make the products smooth and fluffy. Even if consumers want cooling products, distributors and retailers will not order them because of the additional shipping, storage, and more responsibilities. There is an increasing amount of customers who try such freshness and who are using recipes for home-made treatments1. But, even such recipes are asking for essential oils, sugar, glycerin, lanoline, etc. that are far removed from their natural sources. Strong Voices notes that "Approx. A third of body and beauty firms are obviously positioning their products in one direction or another. Nevertheless, certain businesses, as you would imagine, are more conventional than others."

Many individuals who opt for "natural" goods are searching for ingredients whose origins they know, and many businesses now provide the source, as in sodium laurel (coconut) and lanolin (wool), with the scientific name of the ingredient. Tortoise comes from pine trees. Turpentine strengthened her hands and then rubbed her lard (from bacon) to keep her as smooth as I recall. Lard and turpentine might be "natural," but they are good for the skin, and along with that, what is the term "good?" If you find this book in the Eco-Mall, it's fair to say that you're looking for skincare:

(1) is socially safe ("eco-friendly");

(2) does not harm animals (commonly known as the 'cruelty-free');

(3) causes no damage and preferably causes benefit for the human body (it is "nice for the blood").

In light of each of these issues, let us examine "natural" skincare.

Environmentally friendly

The beauty industry never tackles the question of whether goods are environmentally safe. Consumers, including cosmetics, pump 100 tons of contaminants into southern California 's air every day, second only to automotive emissions. These pollutants not only come from spray and aerosol propellants, but also from ethanol, fluorocarbons, acetone, butane, phenols, and xylenes. This works as follows: when the sun shines, these chemicals evaporate, and, with another pollutant, they form ozone, a primary smog component which can lead to headaches, chest pain, and lung loss. This occurs both outside and indoors, which can seriously affect air quality in the homes and offices.

There is a mixture of chemicals called PPCPs (pharmaceutical as well as personal care products), which, as possible environmental pollutants, have until recently received little attention. PPCPs contain all medications, diagnostic agents (e.g., radio compromise media), foods, and other additives, including fragrances, sunscreen agents, and skin anti-aging preparations; PPCPs include all medicines (prescription and over-the-counter). Phthalates join rivers and streams, for example, and are believed to bioaccumulate musk fragrances.3[3] Bugs may be botanic crops cultivated with pesticides and artificial fertilizers that are not environmentally safe, and some may also use genetically engineered plants in the botanical components.

Clear of Cruelty

"Cruel-free" means the products are not tested on animals; often, there is also no animal-derived component in the products. Literally, this means the lack of lanolin (wool), beeswax or honey, milk products, etc. Some labels specifically state that animal ingredients are not available.

Pleasant to the body

Four requirements for "body-friendly" skincare items are suggested:

- ·Toxicity
    - Occlusive
    - Cometographic
    - Efficiency

1. Toxicity

To summarize, phthalates, petrolatum, mineral oils, parabens, propylene glycol, SLS and SLES have been identified. We also asked sunscreens.

Skincare product toxicity (to humans) can be classified into three distinct categories:

a. Carcinogenic ingredients that contribute to cancer

b. Endocrine-disrupting chemicals, which interrupt the hormonal equilibrium of the body and can affect its ability to naturally expand, evolve, or work. Endocrine disruptors can be carcinogenic as well.

c. Allergic, painful, or sensitizing, which means that the users may have allergic reactions or dermatitis by touch (itch, redness, rash, etc.). Individuals with several chemical sensitivities may become very sick if certain of these chemicals become released.

There are many "all" skincare companies that incorporate in their products parabens, SLES, and other ingredients.

A general note on food preservatives: Preservatives are toxic by their very nature. To avoid spoilage, they should be toxic to bacteria, molds, and yeast. Diazolidinyl urea is another preservative used as an alternative to parabens. The use of this preservative in Europe was not banned, but some scholars claim that it is cancerous since it is a donor to formaldehyde. While formaldehyde is a natural chemical in the human body, formaldehyde is considered to be carcinogenic in the gaseous state. From any analysis that we have seen, as it absorbs formaldehyde, Diazolidinyl urea does not form into formaldehyde gas. Nevertheless, Diazolidinyl urea, along with virtually any other preservative, has been shown to induce contact dermatitis when it is used in high amounts or also in low concentrations in people who are highly vulnerable to it. "Raw" goods often claim to not use a preservative. Many produce grapefruit or other citrus extracts of seed oil. As stated in Part I of this show, cosmetic chemists I have said insisting that if they are not treated with a conserving agent, these citrus seeds are rancid, that the preservative is contained in the oil when it is removed, that it conserves the skincare substance in the extract, and that the preservative, in general, is a paraben.

Skincare products are also sold in airless pumps or sprayers in enclosed pots. Such a method of labeling and sourcing is particularly advantageous even if it may dramatically raise the expense of a drug because it removes oxygen and airborn pollutants from the drug and enables the usage of preservatives to be greatly minimized or even removed.

Some relatively few of the large range of suggested cosmetic ingredients pose high-risk individuals, but many use a range of products every day. These risks may add up, or individual ingredients react with each other to make toxic combinations, called synergistic toxicity.

2.Occlusiveness

The skin is the main organ of the body. The heart breathes and the blood, as it were: the "respiratory" blood gives way to chemicals and toxins — respiration in the form of suddenness. Lotions and salves that hide the skin may initially smooth the skin while avoiding moisture, but may actually inhibit individuals' overall health, besides weighing the skin and causing it to become sloppy and tender. Applied skin nutrients that improve the health of the skin may have a positive effect on the whole body as they are absorbed through the skin into the bloodstream. Two key requirements come into play in selecting body-friendly skincare: the goods are not toxic to our skin or our organs so that they don't include occlusive nutrients and toxins.5. The bonus came when the ingredients permitted also balance and feed the skin. Here we deal with ingredients specific to the occlusive and/or comedogenic "normal" skincare.

Look at the "occlusiveness" on the internet, and you can find hundreds of references to occlusiveness and its advantages. The explanation of why businesses profit from occlusion is that it keeps water in the face. When there is no escape from the water, the skin remains soft and moist and sounds good. Picture coating the face in plastic wrap that is serious occlusivity during the day. It will begin to stink there very quickly, as contaminants which usually escape with suddenness and evaporate into the air become stuck between the skin and the material. Now imagine these same toxins can't escape the bloodstream because regular skin breathing is stopped. Where are they going to go? For certain circumstances, they compress under the skin to cause deep blemishes; in certain instances where occlusive lotions are applied in the body for lengthy stretches, it may lodge them in the liver to contribute to the toxic pressure of the body.

Only occlusive salves may be effective for a short amount of time. For starters, if you wish to ascend Mt. Everest or ski at high elevations, where the air is thin and dry, and you are close to the sun, wear a lotion that keeps the waters in the skin is a good idea. It is safe to use a salve for babies with a diaper rash that prevents water away from the skin! There are not permanent conditions for any of us, so over time, therapies that retain water are needed.

This argument can be disputed by traditional beauty experts. Don't head to the Cosmetics Counter Without Specifics: "According to many 'natural' cosmetic firms, mineral petroleum (and petrolatum) comes from crude chemical (oil), is being used in industry to manufacture a metal cutting fluid which can destroy and suffocate the skin by the formation of a chemical picture. It also notes that anti-sweaters "cannot penetrate into the skin." (p. 14). As long as the molecules are small enough to pass through the skin membrane, I hold that anything rubbed onto the skin is absorbed; that is how patches work to deliver medicine. While Begun argues well that crude oil is "natural," I think that it is not my list to make educated choices on the earth-derived substances that we apply to the skin, and crude oil.

It should be remembered that occlusivity levels exist: if an ingredient is occlusive by itself, less occlusive if used in conjunction with non-occlusive ingredients. A small number of beeswax used to emulsify jojoba and water will be much less occlusive than rubbing beeswax on the skin alone. In this context some of the most common occlusive ingredients in "natural" skincare are, in addition to mineral oil and petrolatum:

a)  Wax and another beeswax
b)  Beaver Petroleum
c)  Butter of cocoa
d)  Dimethicalone
e)  Darling
f)  Lanolin
g)  Oil for sunflower and other vegetable oils

3. Comedogen ship

Contrary to occlusive oils like gold, sunflower oil that does not penetrate, comedogenicity refers to a substance 's ability to infiltrate and block pores of the skin. This is extremely troubling in skincare items where obstructed pores can contribute to acne and blackheads. Comedy is the medical term for blackhead, and thus Comedo+Genic is the term "blackhead friendly." Some of the cosmetic glossaries are "non-comedogenic," but that is an incomprehension, while beeswax, mineral oil, zinc oxide (including others). They sit on top of the surface and do not penetrate. Others may be occlusive and (somewhat) comedogenic, like sunflower oil. Below is a fairly comedogenic list of such the "all" cosmetic ingredients6

Most Comedogenic

A shade comedogenic
Not cosmological
Triglyceride Capric / caprylic
Lanolin anhydrous
Allantoin
Butter of chocolate
Advocate in crude
Wax of Beeswax
Acid Lanolic
Acid Capric & Capric
Dimethicone & Cyclomethicone
Oil of Linseed
Raspberry oil
Ethanol
Olive wood
Oil of cocoon

Sweetheart
Corn oil
Peach kernel oil
Sweet almond oil
Jojoba
Kaolin (clay)
Grape seed oil
Oil Mineral (USP)
Glyceryl stearate
Oxybenzone
Hexylene glycol
Lanolin alcohol & butter
Mineral oil, Cosmetic grade,
Panthenol
Oilatum (USP)
Fat of Peanut
Polysorbates Polysorbate
Crop seed Oil
Glycol propylene
Oil of Sesame
Drug SD
Fat of sunflower
Hyaluronate with sodium
PCA Sodium

Tocopherol (vitamin E) Tocopherol
The Sorbitol
Squalene Culture
Dioxide in titanium
Crests

"Note: Only comedogenic ingredients in non-comedogenic formulations may be used with a small percentage to keep pores from being covered in the end solution" (ibid.). The key thing is to look at its relative place in the list of ingredients. If a comedogenic portion is upwards, then it is likely to be present in adequate amounts to block pores. Unfortunately, from the ingredients list, it is difficult to say, for example, that ingredient # 5 constitutes 20% or 2% of the recipe. Thus, if the label says "non-comedogenic," we need to be able to trust the producer.

4. Performance

Let us presume that any skincare company's purpose for being (before or after the profit motive) is to produce products to make the skin feel and look good. Add some more targets, anti-aging, anti-acne, skin smoothing, and most of the bases have been covered. The majority of skincare products, "made" or otherwise, do this by using occlusive ingredients, which keep the skin smooth and "plump."

When, though, we search for the importance of healthy overall skin quality, we must expect more about our skincare.

The Steps You Need to Know About Natural Skin Care and Beauty

Natural skincare has never been more common with anything going green these days. Skincare firms add to their drug list of natural ingredients. Many beauty shops you walk to have natural skincare items in the store. Nevertheless, real natural skincare is more than mere herbal ingredients or home-made treatments for skincare. It's a routine lifestyle.

Good skin treatment and vice versa is a natural beauty. However, more than what you place on your skin is impacted, even whether the drug is normal. Natural skincare involves a lifestyle that always practices healthy habits. If you are eating a poor diet, never exercising and smoking, then no natural product or anybody else will keep your skin young and healthy. The main factor in maintaining a beautiful taint begins from inside. Natural beauty, in other words, is deeper than the skin.

Six factors that affect the look of your skin

1. Diet: What you're getting down. It is as essential as any product that you can put on the skin. A healthy diet full of fruit and vegetables, low in calories, low in bad fat, high in calcium, but plenty of water can do better than any store you find to preserve natural beauty.

2. Physical fitness and sound sleep: skin-friendly workout. It facilitates healthy blood flow to the dermis and gives the skin more oxygen. On the other hand, it's just as important to get enough sleep for perfect skin as we mature. When possible, a typical person will sleep 8 to 9 hours.

3. Environment: the outside and the inside of your skin will affect your skin in many ways. The sky is clearest. UVA / UVB rays will damage our skin to the deeper layers of the collagen. There is no excuse not to cover your skin with all the great sun care solutions. Wind can dry up your skin as well as smog could even leave your skin with a thin filament of dirt, so be sure that your skin remains moisturized and clean. Both heating and air conditioning can affect your skin 's wellbeing.

4. Heredity: In the population, major skin or skin disorders may occur. If your grandma sends you a stunning taint, don't take it for granted. Your skin also needs special treatment. The same applies to skin issues. Don't feel like you can't do it. Following the guidelines and seeking a reliable treatment network, these issues will be strengthened or completely alleviated.

5. Stress: Avoid stress to the fullest extent possible. Too much tension will harm your general wellbeing, including the quality of your skin. Natural skincare involves reducing or removing life tension.

6. Drugs: Certain drugs can affect the skin and can cause rashes, dry skin, or acne. Consult your doctor always if you take medicines that appear to change your skin. Examples include synthetic drugs and certain antibiotics.

Additional guidelines for natural skincare are:

1. Give a dry brush exfoliation to your body.
Exfoliation with dry brush extracts dead skin cells as well as helps to detoxify the skin. Dry brushing also increases the circulation of lymph and blood. The gentle brushing often relaxes the muscles and can help reduce puffiness.

2. Seek to avoid the excess of sugar in your diet.
Eating sugar is one of the major causes of premature aging. Too much blood sugar can contribute to a process called glycation. Glycation occurs where a molecule of glucose (sugar) binds to a molecule of a protein. This breaks the protein molecule and forms a new structure, called advanced glycation end products or Years. Harm to the skin, cartilage, and ligaments by AGE and the lack of elasticity. This leads to shrinkage and wrinkling.

3. Stop things going. Keep things running.
A slow circulation affects your skin by making it hungry for nutrients. You can get swollen, puffy, raise acne, and promote cellulite through inactivity. Therefore, it is very important to take your breaks to walk if you have a career that makes you sat all the time. Chat in the business a couple of runs. Join a club. Enter a club. Get out on Saturday. Get out on Saturday. Good circulation improves your skin and the entire body.

4. Take your digestion again

A healthy digestive system works well for the skin and overall wellbeing. People with skin issues also have stomach problems, such as constipation or imbalances of healthy and poor bacteria.

Start drinking enough water to restore your digestion. Water keeps things in motion, which is always important, through the colon. Then, ensure that you eat ample fiber in the daily diet. In 2002 the Food and Nutrition Board of the National Academy of Sciences proposed that women aged 19-50 years would use 25 grams of fiber a day and over 50 grams of fiber 21 grams. Thirty-eight grams of fiber is recommended for men aged 19 to 50 years. For men over 50 years, 31 grams of fiber must be included in their diet.

Make sure you have all your food foods, coolant, apples with skin, nuts and berries, prunes, peas, legumes, and ground flax seeds in your diet.


5. Eat fats good

The essential fatty acids, such as omega-3 and omega-6, are healthy fats. Without these essential fatty acids, the body cannot survive. Cell membranes, hormones, and other body chemicals require EFA. You protect the heart and battle inflammation. EFA can help dry skin, acne, and eczema patients. Coldwater fish such as sardines or salmon, walnut oil, flaxseed oil, and supplements contain essential fatty acids.


A couple more steps in the natural skincare and beauty program are:

- After every meal, brush your teeth
- Get a weekly facial or shower.
- Treat yourself to total body treatment monthly or more
- Also keep the sun and pollutants from shielding the skin
- Use natural products for skincare

• Be comfortable and trustworthy! A smiling face is always beautiful.


## Natural Cleaning Products: A Simpler, Safer, (and Cheaper) Alternative

For us, natural cleaning has now become a priority. The next time you have been to the grocery store, take a long stroll down the cleaning peninsula. And yeah, now it's taking up a whole island. Take some of the items and read them.

Do you know what these ingredients are?


We realize we do not.

Our very basic rule for cleaning is that we don't buy it and take it home if we don't know what an ingredient is. This applies to food, products of cleaning, anything. If we can't say a word, it's probably a chemical, and it's probably not good for us. Just wonder how people kept their homes tidy in the 1920s? Have they done so with chemicals? Nope. Nope. They used homemade natural cleaning products, some of which are probably right now in your kitchen or office.


Clean up your air, of course.

We don't use air fresheners with canned or plug-in. There are molecules full of surprises. There are endless natural possibilities. There is just a handful here.

Plants that reduce toxic substances are: aloe Vera, ivy, fig-trees, chrysanthemum, Spider, evergreen Chinese, palm, and lily bamboo. Decorate these plants liberally and serve as a natural purifier of the soil.

Beth 's favorite air freshener is vanilla, the number one romantic perfume by guys, by the way. Place in the ceramic bowl one natural tablespoon (not imitation) vanilla extract and placed in a bed. You may want to use more than one room if it is large. When vanilla evaporates, a sweet, soothing fragrance of vanilla wafts into the room. Substitute that day.

The favorite air freshener for Josh is eucalyptus, making the whole house bright and springy. If you have a diffuser, a few drops of eucalyptus oil can be poured into it, freshening the air for hours. We do not actually own a diffuser, so we just use an old sauce pot with a little water on low heat at the bottom. Functions the same way.

Vinegar is the favorite cleaner and so versatile, together with Borax. Mildly acidic white vinegar dissolves soil, soap scum, and shiny surfaces from rough water, but it is soft enough to scrub hardwood floors with a paste.

White vinegar is a good deodorizer to clean the skin. It absorbs smells rather than masks them. We use it to get rid of pet smells, like a bed of our dog Barlow, which often needs good natural cleaning.


Your Home Safe

The following recipe is also my choice and not for cooking. It is a formula for an alkaline natural cleaning agent for all purposes. We use it all: in the shower, in the kitchen, to scrub the tapestries and to clear the dark gun from the walls. It neutralizes smells, dissolves the fat, and eliminates blemishes.

-- one or 40 drops of essential antiseptic oil (thyme, sweet orange, lemon, clove, rose, cinnamon, eucalyptus, birch, rosemary, tea tree, or lavender)

> 1 tablespoon soda baking

➢ 2 Borax tea sticks.

➢ 1 tablespoon detergent oil.

➢ Two hot water-spoons.

In a spray bottle, mix ingredients. Shake to blend before use.

The quality of this natural cleaning agent has been increased. It takes 3 cents to produce when all the ingredients are available. A bottle of all-purpose cleaner purchased from the store costs about $4. We truly feel that this fits better than the shop already buying things. Hmmm, the tough decision here. Hmmm.

This is the perfect cleaner for bottles. Forget what you're buying in shops.

-- 1 c drug brushing
-- 1 c vapor-1 c
-- 1 charcoal with white vinegar
Mix in a bowl of water.

Borax's Mysteries

For those of you not versed in the magic Borax, just go for another stroll down the washing island of your grocery store. A medium-sized cardboard box labeled 'Borax' is available in the laundry department. A complex mineral found in lakes and other deposits of evaporite is also known as sodium borate. It's a cleaning aid that's been used for more than 100 years, but it works for so many more.

Sprinkle on your tapes if you have a problem with your flea, wait a day, and vacuum it up. The fleas eat the Borax, they dehydrate and die.

They most commonly use Borax as a tapestry cleaner. Whenever a wet tap cleaner is borrowed from the food shop, we use 1/2 cup of Borax for a gallon of hot water. Load up the machine instead of the vacuum cleaner that is full of chemicals. Borax disinfects and deodorizes. One-half cup to one gallon of water meets the requirements of a hospital for germicides.

Stop Cleaner Drain Purchase

Drainers use unbelievably powerful chemicals to eat blockages in your pipes. These chemicals then enter our water systems. We are very expensive, and we never need them. Test those recipes. Try them. When they don't work, a chemical drain cleaner isn't going to work either. Perhaps you'll have to snake the drain or employ a plumber if anything else fails.

To disinfect sinks naturally, dump 1 cup of washing soda down a week. Washing soda (sodium carbonate) is a baking soda chemical equivalent (sodium bicarbonate). Soda ash is viewed differently than baking soda. It is caustic so that when we use it, wear gloves. It is available in the washing section of the store.

In clogged drains, bring 1 cup of washing soda into the drainage system as near as possible to the drain. Water will go down within a minute. If you have not backed up any water or have no soda washing yet, pour 1 cup of baking soda and 3 cups of boiling water down the drain.

You should also try a 1/2 cup of baking soda and 1/2 cup of vinegar. Leave in a drainpipe and rinse with hot water for 1 minute.

If it doesn't function, add 1/4 cup of hydrogen peroxide to the drain. Wait, then dive for a few minutes. If required, repeat.

Last but not least, Sells Actinia manufactures a digestive organism that liquidates grapes and waste and reduces or removes smells. For use in drains, pipes, and septic tanks, it is secure. Typically, this drug functions because there is nothing else.

These are only a few of our natural cleaning solutions. Check-in with us, we will periodically post new recipes and ideas. Feel free to email us if you have any concerns or herbal cleaning tips and ideas.

## Safe and Natural Homemade Cleaning Products

The next time you go to the supermarket, homemade cleaning supplies will be on your shopping list. Are not even consumer cleaning products you are looking for? Well, because they can be harmful and because homemade cleaning products are safer and cheaper. Homemade cleaning supplies are usually also made up of things like baking soda, lemon juice, salt, vinegar, sprinkle tubes, olive oil, and bucket. This will purify glass, polish metals, scrub, clean showers, toilets, appliances, wood floors, and everything else you think will work on.

I want to use tea, liquid soap, and vinegar on my walls. Put it in a spray bottle, brush it on the windows, and wipe it clean with a newspaper. You can mix tea tree oil, liquid soap, Limon juice, water, essential oils, and there you have to disinfect areas of the house.

All these approaches are non-toxic and, at the same time, have a safe house for you so that you can't go wrong. You need clean air to breathe too, so try to leave the windows open as much as possible for the ventilation outside your home while you clean your room. If you want a nice, natural scent, consider leaving the coffee ground or lemon peeling in the garbage. These air refreshers can smell fantastic, but you can't breathe in the best stuff. Household cleaning tools are easy and safe to use, and they are guaranteed to clean your home as you read them.



Hello beautiful! If you are a college student or a teacher, these natural homemade beauty tips are useful for any lady. Every day, makeup companies come up with new items, and it is still too overwhelming. I'm not here to slam a beauty brands because a lady uses some of their beauty products, but most of them sell fake promises. Why would a person be knowledgeable and not disturbed? It's not possible at all.

You'll produce the best results with the aid of these simple homemade makeup tips. She uses all these homemade remedies personally and believes that it works. Consumer goods show you instant results, but they last for a limited time. You have to be careful and persistent if you want to see the difference in your face. The most successful and natural DIY makeup tips for women are listed below.

Natural handmade women's makeup tips:
1: For dry skin: When you live in a humid environment, your skin is very dry, and particularly if you have a dry form of skin. Your skin is moisture-free. Your skin needs moisture to stay smooth and natural. Take

two milk tablespoons and add the sweetheart to it. Grab a ball of cotton and add the mixture to your nose. Malai (full cream) can also be used instead of milk. Apply at night, hang tight, and wash your face with cold water for 30 minutes.

2: For oily skin: This skin condition is very difficult, and we sometimes suffer from whiteheads and persistent pimples. 2: For oily skin. The skin develops excess sebum, and therefore pickles are trapped in the pores. The oily skin must also be hydrated. When the skin is too dry, excess oil is produced. Your skin must be clean and clear. You should wear an oatmeal hat, take some oatmeal, and add delicious food. Attach this mask and spray it with the cold water for 30 minutes. Your skin's going to feel cool.

3: For blackheads, the dirt is placed in the pores and causes blackheads when the skin is exposed to dirt and pollution. There are really persistent blackheads. This natural beauty tip can be used to get rid of the dirt. Take a white egg and bring it in honey and lemon. Put all of this on your face and wait for 20-30 minutes. Take a teaspoon of baking powder and apply a little lemon to get rid of the blackheads on the nose. Now put it on your nose and quit for 30 minutes. It'll irritate for a bit, but it's normal. It acts as a cure, and the skin looks so smooth.

4: Instantly gleaming skin: she uses this natural beauty tip to glow instantly. Take that sweetheart and add a few drops on a lemon. Now apply this mask to your face and wash it after 30 minutes with cold water.

5: For dark circles: We live under so much job pressure and tension in a busy world. The lack of sleep and addiction to electronics contributed to the dark circles around the eyes for a long time. Take some almond oil and massage it clockwise and anti-clockwise in the under-eye area. You should take some raw milk and add some rose tea. Add a cotton ball to this combination. You should leave it overnight as well as wash it in the morning with cold water.

6: For lightening the skin: it can tan fast if your skin is exposed to the sun. Potato juice helps the skin to lighten.

7: New skin dewy. Cut some cucumbers and drink it overnight in the cold. Now wash your face early in the morning with this spray. Your skin would look fresh and dewy instantly.

8: for the skin to be moisturized: she washes my face with sugar and always miss the morning cleanser and only brush my face with the sweets. It makes my skin soft and maintains the skin's PH balance.

9: For pimples and acne: You should get rid of the dirt once a week with Multani mitti 's face and rose water. If you have particularly dry skin, add some honey or a few drops of coconut oil. Apply this kit for 20 minutes and wipe the cool water on your nose.

10: For facial hair: hormonal changes could contribute to the growth of the beard. If the hormones fluctuate, it disturbs the equilibrium and contributes to hair growth in the chin and jaw regions. A facial bag of besan (gram flour) sugar and lemon can be used. Apply this pack for twenty minutes and wash it with cold water. Use this pack twice a week to see the results faster. It does not remove all hair but lightens the hair and grows gradually.

There were some highly powerful and natural makeup tips for ladies.

She is still using these homemade natural beauty tricks and have seen a big improvement in skin health. You have to make sure you have a balanced diet, and it won't make any difference, regardless of whether you do outside if you don't take care of your food. You will eat the right things. The secret to caution. Don't expect the miracles instantly. Whoever guarantees you an instant response would definitely sell the false goods. It takes a lot of time and extra work to have a safe and beautiful skin before you are actually born with it.

The only thing you can do for your skin and your body is to go normal. The skin's going to thank you later. These pure organic beauty tips have no side effects, and she promises that these home remedies are the perfect option for all skin types. Keep your body hydrated and follow these treatments so that your skin is smooth and light.

## CLEANING RECIPES

### Natural Cleaning Recipe

This is shocking that more people are wasting money on vitamins and other nutritional products. And they do not care twice about their home use when it comes to domestic cleaners filled with harmful chemicals. The irony is that you can not only improve your health by combining your own natural cleaning ingredients but also save a huge amount of money.

As your heritage your genome from parents, soon after conception, you begin to map what researchers call your epigenome during fetal development. This mechanism is to turn genes on or off based on the environment. Scientists believe that these genetic variations can be reversed after birth and that these genetic modifications affect the domestic cleaners with toxic chemicals.

In other words, chemical substances can cause a gene to be switched on. The result is that you can indeed have a foot from your hand, but a whole spectrum of genes is responsible for the growth of the entire foot, and so what you have instead is called a tumor. There are many causes of cancer, but most are due to epigenetic alterations in our DNA, modifications, or defects in our epigenome.

Below is a simple tapestry cleaning formula.
- ❖ 4 cups of soda or maize starch
- ❖ Eucalyptus 35 drops of mineral oil
- ❖ 30 drops of Essential Lavender Oil
- ❖ 25 drops of liquid Rosewood oil

In a bowl, place baking soda and add the essential oils. Shake the clumps and blend properly.

Sprinkle the powder on the carpet from a shaker or jar, and quit to clean for about 15 minutes.

Many people are investing a lot of time and resources on diets, wellness centers, and other self-enhancement practices. Nevertheless, they seem to be unaware of the risks when it comes to hazardous substances in their houses. You may be surprised to know that many chemicals contain hormone disruptors, like estrogen imitation. Hormone estrogen allows the body to retain fat more efficiently since estrogen levels in a woman rise during pregnancy.

## Organic Colon Clean Recipe

While the web provides different types of organic colon cleaning recipes, the safest and easiest one uses pure sea salt. If you've ever searched the internet for a clean recipe of the organic colon, the results may have flooded you. This is a big challenge to take down only a tiny amount of them. This is why this basic formulation is given. Take a spoonful of pure sea salt and blend in 8 cups of sugar.

If you do this job in the winter season, you can use tidy snow. Using the Muslin or some other fie fabric as long as the salt has dissolved. Now gradually and absolutely drink this saltwater. Initially, you might feel like throwing up, but you have to be patient. Do not forget that you have to clean up your colon. Only relax or spend a few minutes cycling, while the salt starts responding. You will feel anxious in about 30 minutes to use the washroom.

It ends the colon cleaning process. You would be able to go 15-20 trips to the toilet. Be careful to observe, and you will notice that your bowel movements are smoother. Repeat this 2-4 times a year. Pregnant women should never attempt to cleanse their colon or take medications because they may damage the fetus. You should call a doctor for issues with your indigestion or constipation.


Nontoxic Household Cleaning Recipes


Green cleaning involves using items that do not harm the atmosphere or your babies. Backing soda, white vinegar, and liquid soap are ingredients found in natural washing recipes. You will need to buy certain items: a pad, washcloth or sponge of cotton, cotton rag (minimum lint), and a 16-ounce spray bottle.

Green cleaning receipts to make non-toxic household cleaners are listed below:

Cleaner tub and sink (soda and liquid soap)

On porcelain fittings, spray baking soda. Rub dirty rag. Add a few drops of liquid to the cloth, Murphy's soap for washing. Rinse well to prevent a hazy image from going.

Cleaner window and mirror (water and white vinegar)

In a spray bottle, put 1/4 cup of white vinegar and fill with water to the rim. Air mist. Water mist. Rub a lint-free rag of cotton. Using a sponge to scrub with hot water for outside walls, with a few drops of liquid Murphy or castile soap inside it. Rinse thoroughly and dry squeegee.

Cleaner linoleum floor (water and white vinegar)

Mop with 1/2 cup mixture of vinegar in a warm water bucket. The odor of vinegar is dissipated soon after the ground dries.

Cleaner toilet bowl (baking soda and soap liquid)

Inside the cup spray baking soda, like you can spread some water. Add a few drops of liquid soap. Scrub the outside surfaces with a bowl of the toilet and finish with a rag sprinkled with baking soda.

Cleaner for both uses (liquid soap)

Using the liquid soap of Murphy to eliminate woodworking, tile, and linoleum stains. Fill in a damp wash pan with a few drops of liquid soap and massage the surface easily.

Cleaner oven (soda and tea bakery)

Mix 1 cup of baking soda to make a paste with enough water. Apply the paste on the surfaces of the oven and let it stand a bit. To wash most items, using the scouring brush. A spatula or a bread knife may be put under major food deposits. This recipe will take more scrubbing, but it is not harmful to you, your children, and the environment. Commercial oven cleaners are highly irritating. Do not use this cleaner in self-cleaning furnaces!

Cleaner wash (soda restaurant, white vinegar, and hot water)

Drain 1/2 cup of baking soda, then 1/2 cup of vinegar. Let it fizz for a couple of minutes. Then pour a teakettle of boiling water in. Repeat if necessary. Using a plunger if the clog is persistent. Use a mechanical snake for very stubborn clogs. This formula prevents small obstructions and helps avoid potential obstructions.


Copper purification (white vinegar, salt, and water)

Mix the same vinegar and salt pieces (each tablespoon) and add a rag to the soil. Make sure to clean afterward vigorously with water, or it will corrode. Don't use this lacquered cleaner!

Use this green cleaner to create homemade cleaning products that are good for you, your children, and the world.


Home Cleaning Recipes with Vinegar


Although many cleaning products are hard and aggressive, damage the surfaces of your house and are far from eco-friendly Where is the point of taking too much money out of the purse if you can use basic home-cleaning vinegar recipes? That's right! That's right! Simple vinegar can clean your house at less expensive and is also an option for green cleaning.

There are a lot of vinegar cleaning supplies at home, and if you find out what you need for every spot in the building, cleaning is better than you can imagine. Some cleaning products use white vinegar as it is less toxic and doesn't harm the bathroom or kitchen surfaces. This is nice to extract hot water or soap from the appliances and is also perfect at washing hardwood floors. You don't have to fear that the flooring will be ruined, and it is not acidic enough. Vinegar home cleaning products can also be used as deodorizers or as softeners for the clothing. You will slowly replace a lot of your shopping cart products. You wouldn't have to worry about the scent of vinegar because you won't feel it anymore once it's dry.

One of the most popular recipes for home vinegar is the mixing of equal proportions of vinegar and water in a sprayer bottle. You have your own cleaning product which works on most of your house's surfaces. It's perfect for countertops, walls, and other quickly dusty kitchen surfaces. The floors along the outside of the toilet can be cleaned in the bathroom. For example, if you want to clear more stubborn dirt like deposits on shower walls, remove the solution from the spray, heat it, and then apply it to the dirty surface. Leave for 10 to 15 minutes, and the stains should certainly be gone.

Most home cleaning vinegar requires the use of undiluted vinegar. It certainly has a higher cleaning capacity. You can use simple vinegar to scrub the inside of the toilet. It removes blemishes and dirt and also removes harmful bacteria. Pour undiluted vinegar into the toilet and scrub it with a brush toilet. Use a pumice stone for stubborn hard water deposits. Dashing heads that are obstructed by hard water deposits are particularly difficult to clean. Luckily, home cleaning vinegar recipes may also solve this issue. In a plastic bag, add some vinegar and place the head of the shower there. Cover the bag with a rubber band and remove the head for a few hours. The alcohol is going to do great things. Undiluted vinegar can also easily be used to supplement synthetic clothing softener. It's great for sensitive skin patients.

Green Cleaning Your Bath Fixtures - Naturally!

How else would you buy cleaning supplies which are toxic and chemical-charged if you invested in high-quality baking equipment or other luxurious plumbing products? Over time, the bathrooms can be damaged by porcelain, rubber, steel, and plastics that inflict scratching or chipping. Above all, talk of what your grandma did-she made just as effective her own cleaning products. But we like to think of this phenomenon as "green cleaning" in this day and age.

The cleaning products you make are actually non-toxic and probably better, but you need more time you need to sit down and batch yourself, so this solution will be more effective as all the other items in the store today that are less environmentally friendly.

I would like to share some of the best homemade cleaning products with you – liquids, pastes, and stain removers in which you are able to make yourself – without harmful chemical cleaning products. Try this on your bathrooms, and we are confident you 're going to want to switch for good!

Basic products for washing your luxurious plumbing goods

It is easy and can be done in no time to create natural cleaning products for use on your fine, luxury plumbing products. There are, though, certain items that should still be in the cupboard:

Baking soda: only as a natural deodorizer, this functional non-toxic replacement filter works perfectly to eliminate stains on your buttons, lever, and bath fittings that can be hard to clean. This is naturally abrasive and is one of the green cleaners most effective.

Lemons: Use all your luxury plumbing products as a natural bacterial combatant and acid cleanser for toilet and sink areas.

Borax: A all-in-one cleaner, sodium borate purifies walls and surfaces, deodorizes, and eliminates mold production in most of the toilets and the showers and walls. Borax:

Vegetable-based (Castile) soap: Available as a bath, a flake, or a tube, all premium filling items and fittings are washed.

Distilled white vinegar: nearly instantly extracts soap scum, dirt, mildew, and dried wax on your finest baths.

Tea tree oil: Good for bathroom deodorization and disinfection. This easily slices the expensive plumbing goods by mold and mildew.

Hydrogen peroxide: A chemical antiseptic that works best in bathrooms to prevent the growth of dangerous bacteria.

Each of these products can efficiently clean luxury products on its own, but when combined, they become super sturdy green cleansers, you will use them again and again. You can find useful recipes on the internet, and these are just some of the best recipes for keeping your toilets and baths closely clean.

Cleaner toilet bowl: Blend 1/4 cup baking soda with 1 cup vinegar. Load in the basin of the toilet and let it cool. After a couple of minutes, powder, and scrub with a toilet brush (1).

Mix 1/2 tablespoon of soda with a touch of fluid soap and two cups of hot water. Shake to blend and remove all ingredients (2).

Scrubbing paste: Mix sufficient soap with 1/8 cup of baker soda to form a creamy mix. Rinse the newly washed area vigorously with water after the stain or coating has been scrubbed and removed (3).

A common approach to fine porcelain washing

It may be difficult to clean the porcelain bath fixtures – if you are using the regular items from the store, you will be shocked. Porcelain may be glazed and unglazed, and the color of the cleaning substance has become known as unglazed bits.

Mix equal parts of vinegar and warm water to one solution if you notice hard-water scum on some of your luxurious plumbing products or bath fittings. Then vigorously wash the area and rinse with water. Or, to clean your bathroom fittings commonly and thoroughly, simply mix a tablespoon of detergent with a gallon of hot water.

Remove Chemicals-Go for good Non-Toxic.

Purchase spray bottles, buckets or pails, and glass jars for the next clean-up to keep your newer pastes, cleaners, and mixtures convenient.

And whether you want or not to make your own eco cleaning products, you will add even more to the environment. In addition to paper towels, try cleaning with reusable rags, made of old cotton-based clothing that you can no longer wear to clean the ropes, handles, and other luxury plumbing products. This way, you generate less waste by recycling everything in the building.

There are many ways to clean your bathrooms environment and greening is just one of them. This small amount removes many problems, such as inserting chemicals and potential threats to children and animals into the air you breathe. For comparison, the best return on your investment is the pleasure of meeting millions in people around the world who want the greenway to clean up their luxurious plumbing goods and bath fixtures.

Green Cleaning Recipes That Keep Your Home Clean and Green!

Green cleaning recipes are not harmful and can be quickly packed. You, the world, and your wallet are fine.

The kitchen also has the most eco cleaning products. All you have to do is mix and match a green cleaning recipe, which can achieve optimal results without harming the environment.

Fresheners Air

Most artificial air fresheners contain toxic additives, which can decrease the health and atmosphere of an individual. They pollute indoor air without knowing it. Place baking soda in the refrigerator and trash bins to reduce odor and avoid polluting indoor air.

You should also disinfect and deodorize the mattress with baking soda. Just sprinkle freely and allow the carpet to living for an hour.

Cleaner Wash

Sink small bubbles, by dumping baking soda into the sink, and then add vinegar. Allow it to fizz for a few minutes, then dump the boiling water into the sink. Continue the cycle until the barrier is loosened.

Cleaner Oven

Baking soda, mix salt, and hot water and make a paste and keep the oven clean. Add the paste to the surface and hold the paste for a couple of minutes or even overnight. Rinse the surface of the mud. Scrub the floor.

Hardwood floors vacuum cleaner

In 1 gallon of warm water, mix the cup of distilled white vinegar. To sweep the wood floor, using a wet mop. Water rinse but do not flood to allow for fast drying.

Polish

Mix 5 ml of lemon oil in olive oil of 250 ml for polishing the furniture. Rinse with a cool, dry rag in the furniture.

To be polished, add a liter of mineral oil and a few drops of lemon oil, melt 1/8 cup of paraffin wax in a double boiler. Add to the floor before polishing, let it dry.

Using these eco cleaning tips, your home can smell clean and fresh without polluting the atmosphere!

## FOOD RECIPES

### Healthy Eating Food

If you'd like to improve the health and wellbeing, exercise and eat a healthy diet are important. You will also ensure that the food you select is one that is called preventive. Today heart failure and issues with elevated blood pressure tend to increase, and unhealthy lifestyle habits are one of the key reasons. Healthy food options are required to reduce the risk of cardiovascular and circulatory issues.

A large proportion of the US population thinks a healthy diet should be boring and bland. That is definitely not the case since safe food preferences provide a wide variety of tasty alternatives. For balanced food recipes, these ingredients are utilized to produce tasty meals that are as elegant, savory, and enticing as those richer and less balanced menus for 5-star restaurants worldwide.

When it comes to healthy food choices, the main guideline is a balanced diet. In fact, your heart appreciates as much as the rest of your body, the most beautifully healthy diet. A healthy diet includes fresh fruit and vegetables; natural whole grains; high-fiber food; high-protein and other maggot ten foods; fish and seafood; and milk products that are 1% or fat-free.

These are the big hips, Sodas, Candy, and Potato chips.

These addictive sodas and snack foods are some of the poorest nutritional choices. Besides sugars and salt, all of these contain hundreds of extra calories for the body. The best results here are two tips to ensure that your diet plan for healthy eating remains ongoing.

* Where the label contains sugar, sugar is contained in sucrose, maize syrup, glucose, maltose, fructose, dextrose, honey, or concentrated fruit juice. When the sugar is one of the first four ingredients on the label, the sugar quantity is very high. These are the ones you would like to stop.

Understanding the fats and awareness

Unsaturated fats do not add to the amount of cholesterol as saturated and Trans fats may. As part of the balanced eating plan, you can continue to use small quantities of unsaturated fats.

Choose Meats Carefully

Know how to pick the finest meat cuts and make sure you use skinless, sliced poultry products. A balanced food program involves meat processing without the use of saturated or trans fats.

- 3 ounces of cooked meat contains about 70 mg cholesterol.
- The AHA (American Heart Association) recommends a maximum of 6 oz of meat, fish, marine, or poultry.
- Beef classified as "choice" or "select" is leaner than those classified as "prime."
- The leanest cuts of Beef are sirloins, chucks, rounds, and loins and should be used in healthy foods.
- Always select the lean or extra lean beef varieties.
- Long chops and tenderloin sections are the leanest pork cuts.

Remove any visible fat before cooking from meat and poultry products.

- If you have poultry in your diet, eating white meat rather than dark meat is your healthiest choice.
- Processed meat has large quantities of chemical substances, sodium, and saturated fats and should be removed from your diet.
- The fat content of the duck and goose is much higher than chicken and turkey meat.
- Limit the grilling, baking, or broiling cooking methods.
- Stop animal meats due to elevated cholesterol levels on the safe food diet plan.

One by country and two by sea

Fish or seafood should be included in your healthy diet at least twice a week.

- Fish are low in saturated fats; even fatty fish have low saturated fats.
- Oily fish have high levels of omega-3 fatty acids, such as herring, salmon, and trout. The risk of heart failure and heart problems can be that of Omega 3.
- Exchange breaded fried fish recipes for healthy food recipes instead of baked, grilled, or broiled fish.

You can now get wild seafood right at your door. For you, it's much better than farmed seafood.

Fatless Dairy Products

- Restrict your diet from the quantity of whole fat milk products and 2% of all fat dairy products.
- Make a step-by-step transition from whole or 2% milk to fat-free products.
- In your healthy eating selection, use fat-free or low-fat cottage cheese. You can also use other fat-free or fat-free cheese products such as ricotta or skim milk mozzarellas.

Decreased use of partially hydrogenated vegetable oils reduces the consumption of trans fat.

- Instead of shortening liquid vegetable oil should be used when developing a balanced diet system.
- Good food meals should use substitutes of heart-healthy soft margarine for certain butter sticks.
- Limit cookies, crackers, cakes, muffins, and other fried foods with fats specified on the label that are partially hydrogenated or saturated.

Cut the counts of cholesterol in the balanced food diet.

- Your total daily cholesterol intake should not exceed 300 mg.
- Chicken eggs should be used for a free ranch in place of other varieties.
- Replace egg whites in preparation of healthy food recipes with whole eggs. In egg whites, there is no cholesterol.
- you must avoid the most.

Reduce the sodium and reduce the chance of heart and stroke
Too much sodium or salt increases the likelihood of high blood pressure, heart attack, and strokes.

The maximum salt in your healthy diet should not exceed 2300 a day.

- Select foodstuffs on the list that have the lowest sodium content.
- Search for "sodium-reduced" or "heart disease, sodium-free" products.
- Limit the use of standard soy sauce, steak sauces, pickles, and olives with high amounts of sodium.
- You can replace your salt with salt-free or natural herb seasoning mixtures.
- Chili peppers and citrus fruits will add free salt and zest to food.
- Rinse and drink your cans with feta cheese, capers or tuna, and salmon. It helps to eliminate excess sodium.

Using Chase Away High Cholesterol Fiber and Oat Bran
Soluble fiber applied to your diet will help you reduce the cholesterol levels in the blood. It also reduces your chance of developing colon / rectal cancers and diabetes. It is advised to use 25-35 grams of dietary fiber

(both soluble and insoluble) every day. A good rule of thumb is to allow 14 grams of dietary fiber in your daily diet per 1,000 calories.

- Oat bran, Oatmeal, peas, barley, rice bran, beans, berries, citrus fruits, and apples are all high in soluble fiber.
- Insoluble fiber is available in whole wheat bread, cereals and bran; coco; apple skin; beets; sprouts in Brussels; turnips; carrots and chocolate flower;
- Replace fiber-rich food with fiber-rich ones. You can substitute the regular white bread for a whole-grain type, for example, and replace white rice for brown rice.
- You eat raw vegetables and fresh fruit rather than frying them first.

Write the Healthier, Happier Heart Labels kit.

When you read the packets and product labels, it will quickly become a daily habit. Then you can decide in an educated way what you want to use in your balanced diet. You will be on the way to a healthy, safer lifestyle when you pick the food wisely.

The Essentials of a Healthy Food Recipe

And more individuals than ever on the Internet, users will select from hundreds of recipes. Naturally, most of the recipes that you find online are not actually safe. Most of them are actually quite unhealthy. But, that just doesn't mean that from time to time, you can't try more. It's nice for you to have fun food once in a while, physically, so don't get used to eating high-fat, unhealthy meals daily. Search for balanced online meals that can be added to the daily meal schedule instead.

A balanced diet will also be wonderful.

Most of the negative raps that healthy eating has received through the years are that it's not as good as enjoying the same diet that everybody else loves. After all, we all know it can't be perfect nutritious food, right?

Nothing could be more than the facts. As many, if not more, delicious, healthy foods as junky ones are available. The cooking includes much of what makes a meal healthy. Even a pie isn't so good when it is correctly cooked. The same concept applies to healthy recipes as to junk food. The essence of a perfect meal is the planning and processing of the ingredients.

Good Meals-New Ingredients Feel

If you're looking for healthy food and better meals for your family, you have to start with the ingredients at the beginning. Some of the better food products are nuts, vegetables as well as whole grains. To get the most delicious ingredients, you simply need to get the freshest food. Take the time for fruit and vegetable shopping. Don't just take your first pepper or lettuce head in front of you. Take note of your vegetables and choose the freshest ones you can find. New vegetables are healthier for you and make the meal taste much better.

Spice Up Stuff

Many claims that balanced foods are fragile. When you turn anyone away with a plate of raw vegetables, then it may be accurate, but planning will also make a better food taster. Don't think about mixing and using herbs and other ingredients. Cut green and red peppers can be mixed into almost any appetizing entry. You can discover nutritious recipes that everybody enjoys if you're searching for opportunities to bring a little flavor to your meals. New garlic is another perfect way to give your meals taste, and it's still really good. But don't go for spices or garlic overboard because they can bother the stomach of certain men. Moderation is best used.

Origin of lean protein

You may believe that healthy eating is associated with vegetarianism. Naturally, if you take a balanced approach to your eating and make sure you get enough protein, you will not go wrong. Yet if you're patient, you don't have to become a vegetarian. Not all healthy recipes require you to completely skip the meat. Most of the time, they allow you to select meats and poultry in a smarter way.

Try to find leaner cuts when serving beef. T-Bones are a popular beef cut but loaded with fats that are unhealthy. You can serve a healthy meal that is low in fat by switching to the slightest cut, like round steak. Make sure you go skinless with chicken and prefer white meat over black. Just purchasing skinless chicken and choosing abreast of the chicken over dark meat will help you cook a nutritious meal of far less fat than the regular beef or chicken eaten by most people.

Check for healthy recipes

If you choose a nutritious meal for your children, select a good meal. A recipe with a selection of foods is more likely to contain ample nutrients. One way to make nutrient-dense foods is by coloring them. You will certainly receive tons of vitamins, minerals, and nutrients from multiple sources by selecting foods in varying colors. And eating a variety of foods will make your family want healthy, delicious food.

You don't have to be fancy or a master chef to create a healthy meal recipe for your next meal. Bear in mind the value of serving nutritious food and making good, thoughtful decisions about all the ingredients you use in your dishes.

Recall that any attempt will not be a success when you seek new recipes. When you first try health food recipes, you may find it doesn't work the way you expect. Don't give up entirely on the recipe. You may boost it by following any of the tips mentioned in this chapter or by including a safe supplement such as Profect in your recipes. Profect contains just the right amount of protein and virtually no calories from Protica. There are some other Protica protein supplements you can use.

Adding the right spices and some fresh ingredients could make this recipe perfect. A lifetime effort would be safe food. And the master chefs on tv make a meal that does not go well every now and then. Keep on preparing nutritious meals, and the relatives will be rushed to get back and see what is for dinner before you know it.



Risotto is one of the super tasty food-cooking restaurants that many people love to order and enjoy, but are much too afraid to attempt and cook at home. She assumes these alerts are about how the danger can continually be pushed and hovered around which people are switched off, which, by the way, is not completely accurate; you can't really patch it and forget it, but you don't have to save it. A friend is not an experienced risotto builder, but surely not a slave driver my recipe below! It only takes 25 minutes to finish, and you can chop a salad or putter in the kitchen during the cooking time.

In a restaurant or anywhere else, she 'd not eat risotto myself, unless she could see precisely what was going on since risotto (like lasagna and smooth soups!) is one of those dishes that an incredible number of unpleasant things will disappear almost uncovered. It's funny because she remembers reading an item that appeared to be written in the NY Times only last year about how a risotto order can be disappointed in a restaurant. She just went to find the post online. This turned out years ago! (Where's the time. The Cliff Note explanation is that calorie counting isn't an effective way to try to check your weight because sometimes fitness professionals don't want to do it right. The risotto was taken as it was one of the dishes for which four healthcare professionals were asked to "determine" the fat and calorie value. As cited in the paper, "The findings were all over the place: a risotto platter was estimated to contain between 500 and 1000 calories and 25 to 70 grams fat. When separate labs tested the dishes, 1,280 calories and 110 grams of fat were contained in the risotto." WHAT? One thousand two hundred eighty calories and 100 g of fat?!?!? She is no fan of food counting (points, calories, fat grams, etc.), but for any single dish, that's a totally ridiculous amount of calories and fat grams. No more risotto restaurant for me!

Unless you know calories and fat grams, most risotto is made with poor Arborio rice nutrients and fiber. For the genuine creaminess aspect, she uses some Arborio rice, but she also adds super-healthy quinoa with lots of veggies and zeroes butter or cream. But if you want to make it extremely healthy, you could only completely eliminate the Arborio rice and use just the quinoa as it has a fabulously creamy texture when cooked slowly. (If you are struggling to extract Arborio rice, give me a note to tell me what's happening!) In the meantime, there's a safe, simple to convenient whole food recipe that doesn't take hours in the kitchen ... just 25 minutes!

Serve ingredients: 6

Three cups of organic fruits (e.g., Pacific Natural Foods)

One leek, trimmed stems, cut into 1-inch parts, thoroughly washed.

Two whole carrots, sliced into bits.

Two tablespoons of extra virgin olive oil (like the Kirkland line of Costco)

Three garlic cloves, hacked.

Sea salt (as the Kirkland brand of Costco) to taste
1/2 cup of rice Arborio
1/2 cup of cinema
Black pepper freshly baked, to taste.
One tablespoon of thyme dry
Chardonnay 1/4 cup
Organic tomatoes one can (15.5 ounces) (such as Muir Glenn)

2 cups semi-thawed, frozen maize kernels

Toppings optional:

Parmigiano Reggiano shredded 1/2 cup (as Costco 's brand Kirkland)

1/2 cup of pecans (like Costco brand Kirkland), transformed into "crumbs" by a food processor

1. Bring the broth to a boil over high heat in a small saucepan. Reduce heat to keep it constantly simmering.

2. In a food processor, put leeks and shred. Match with vegetables. Vegetables. Place aside. Set aside.

3. Heat the oil over medium-high heat in a large, heavy cup, add garlic, and bake for 30 seconds. Add sliced carrots and leeks and sauté for 3-4 minutes or tenderly. Only season vegetables with oil. Add the rice and quinoa to the casserole and simmer for about 2 minutes, stirring continuously.

4. Sprinkle thyme over the cereals. Add Chardonnay; whisk to evaporate wine. In the pot with the beans, add 1/2 cup of hot broth and the tomatoes, stirring continuously. Start adding 1/2 cup of broth at a time and stir periodically it until liquid has also been drained, until each 1/2 cup of water is added. Cook the grains for around 25 minutes over medium heat or until all the moisture is absorbed, stir regularly so that the grains don't stay with the bowl.

5. Stir in the semi-thawed corn seeds and cover the pan and allow the risotto to sit for 15 minutes until serving.

6. Alternatively: top rice with cheese or pecans shredded (or both!).

Crunchy granola hippie products is no longer smoothies. They are in sidewalk cafes and are sold in 6 packages in the grocery store. However, smoothies are easy to make at home and can also be healthier if you grow them. One of the best reasons for starting to drink smoothies is when you are likely to skip breakfast.

The main meal of the day is breakfast, yet millions of people go out with a coffee thermos and a full to-do list. Your body needs fuel for proper functioning. Your brain needs energy for proper thinking. Smoothies are a perfect way to make a tasty dessert of great nutrients. They can be exchanged instantly and conveniently. What else can you like to have a great breakfast?

My list here is as follows: juice (I mix it), full-flax yogurt, flax seeds, super green powder, coconut milk powder, flaxseed oil, and wheat germ.

You can begin with the powder of juice, green food, yogurt, and the coconut milk and use flax seeds, protein powder as well as other ingredients. I recommend a powdered super green mix as it easily mixes and digests very fast. (I often mix it with a cup of juice as well as take a green shot to pick me for a mid-afternoon!) Moreover, it's cheaper than other regimes of vitamins as all the nutrients you need are shot in one. I really like to add vanilla protein powder and chocolate powder, although they add more protein, including omega-3 fatty acids, plus a very creamy and pleasant taste of the chocolate milk powder! Okay, now that your basic ingredients are there!

For many reasons, smoothies are good for you, but two in particular. One: smoothies incorporate readily available liquid nutrients. This means that you immediately get the nutrients in a protein-rich form. Second: on the go, they 're great healthy food. Let's face it for a fast-paced society, and we require better food. Before you go, put another USD 5 billion a star buck-try to make your own smoothies and feel the super green difference in food!

Smoothie without the use of a blender

Yellow fluffy

1 cup of juice of an orange (to taste)
1 cup of plain or yogurt of vanilla
One tb of a super green powder energy

One tb of powdered coconut milk
2-3 ice cubes (helps to blend and hold cold)
Place ingredients in a tight-deck container and shake or whisk vigorously.
Dream of raisins
2 cups of the juice of grape (to taste)
Dust with 1 cup with vanilla powder
1 tsp of super green powder strength
1 tsp of powdered coconut milk
2-3 cubes of ice (helping to blend and hold frozen ingredients)
Place the ingredients in a jar with close deck and shake or whisk vigorously.

This one is smooth and sweet.
Zest of Cranberry Lemon
1 cup of juice of cranberry (to taste)
1 cup of plain or yogurt of vanilla
1 tsp of super green powder strength

1 tsp with orange juice

2-3 cubes of ice (helping to blend and hold frozen ingredients)

Place the ingredients in a jar with close deck and shake or whisk vigorously.

It is a fantastic and genuine zinger when it's heavy!

Smoothie recipes with your mixer

This is easy before work, and you can do it.

Allow enough for your mates to share too!


Fun Apple Banana

One taste of apple juice

1 cup of plain or yogurt of vanilla

1 tsp of super green powder strength

1 tsp sprout

One big (with or without peel) cored apple

One mature banana

2-3 ice cubes

Mix the ingredients and eat cold

This one turns out to be very nasty and good! I have a mild texture and a wonderful nutty flavor with the wheat germ.

Banana coconut cream

One-half cup of fresh water filtered

Powder of half cup of coconut milk

1 cup of plain or yogurt of vanilla

1 tsp of super green powder strength
2 tsp flax grains

One mature banana

Half a half-cup (optional, but good)

2-3 ice cubes

Mix the ingredients and eat cold
Okay, are you prepared for a warm, fluffy, coconut, and that's very good for you? Try this recipe! Try this recipe!

I use fruit for this, and I hold the fridge, try it-it's simple. The next time the bananas, blueberries, as well as strawberries (or any other fruit) go bad, simply peel and freeze into a bag. Then I use these chunks all year round for smoothies! It replaces the ice and gives great taste and texture to your smoothies.

The frozen delight of slushy

1 cup of 2% milk
1 cup of plain or yogurt of vanilla
1 tsp of super green powder strength
2 tsp flax grains

One cup of fruit frozen.
One mature banana
Powder 2 tsp cocoa milk
Seed oil 1 tbsp flax
One vanilla extract spray

Mix the ingredients and eat cold

Sanitary bloody marriage

2 cups of tomato/juice of vegetables

1 tsp of super green powder strength

One-fourth cup of celery leaves

2 -3 fresh leaves of basil

2-3 ice cubes


Mix ingredients and drink in ice, along with fresh celery sticks.

You now have all these tasty options to add a super green drink to your morning-what do you expect.




---

## Good Food Good Health - Garlic

For several years, garlic has had significant health benefits and is also considered as 'antibiotic' by definition, but people are hesitant to consume fresh garlic because its delicious odor leaves their breath or is excreted in pores. Garlic has this effect because it's not metabolized, but absorbed by the lining of the stomach.

It has now become clear that the use of a good quality allicin supplement (the active ingredient of garlic) gives you equal efficacy, and naturally, you may use the odorless variety because that garlic is aged and detoxified and then deodorized.

I adore garlic, and I'm excited for some kind of savory stuff, however as the family minority have taken odorless capsules in order to preserve calm. I think garlic is one of the few products that everybody has a view on; either you love it, or you hate it!

Literally, my daddy-in-law, Joe, eats raw cloves every day, perhaps one of the reasons he was not poor health in his 1980s. Joe comes from Poland, where garlic was used for years and years for health reasons, especially consumed against influenza, but often topically rubbed onto the soils of his feet to shield him from cold and many others.

But yes, the odor problem came to me in the maternity center when I had the older daughter, the nurses couldn't believe that after visiting us, the odor lingered and they told him they 'd worry that the babies on the ward would get upset. Of course, he was a little insulted, but more ashamed, though we had raised the subject before, thank you for this time. He still uses garlic, but he does not take an odorless daily supplement every day.

To date, garlic has been researched in various forms, and it appears that its benefits tend to grow. For some years now, the biggest reason I've used garlic is the impact it has on the body's immune system.

Our bodies could do a little better of all the tension of today's society. The antioxidant compounds found in garlic come from sulfur-containing selenium and germanium, which improve the immune system.

This is this method that enables rid the body of free radicals which are known to be associated with aging, tumor development, and atherosclerosis. Garlic, in its raw state, is considered to be one of your natural killing cells' most powerful boosters. This alone would allow lovers of non-garlic to change the mind.

Work has shown that garlic-allicin is an outstanding natural antimicrobial and can deter a significant range of infectious species. These antibiotic properties could be highly active against infections of yeast, fungi, and viruses.

Garlic is also great for your heart because it has the properties to fight 'bad' cholesterol. Today we all know that high-density HDL lipoprotein, which is not dangerous but LDL lipoprotein, is certainly because it can be oxidized by dangerous free radicals. The antioxidant properties of garlic help to reduce free radical damage.

Garlic is natural aspirin because it can help prevent the clumping of red blood cells. Naturally, garlic keeps the blood thin that is necessary to prevent strokes and heart attacks, so those who take regular garlic benefit from the very same as aspirin but without any other risks, but they should not be taken instead of prescribed medication.

Garlic is often beneficial to coronary circulation and has shown itself to increase circulation in the peripheries of the body, which is incredibly helpful, particularly because it is always difficult to get adequate exercise.

Research is still being carried out to determine the effect of garlic on cancer cells, and the findings on mice look promising. To date. This is genuinely inspiring.

I hope you 're not a garlic lover, so you've got a good idea of the benefits of eating or at least taking a supplement. You will not only benefit from your safety, but you will also benefit from knowing that you are free from vampires!!

Garlic has long been written about. 22 Egyptian garlic cures were contained on papyrus from the 16th century BC. Because of its antibacterial properties, it was also the reason Vikings were not going on long sea voyages without garlic. African missionaries have found the garlic has prevented dysentery successfully.

In fact, my granddad was growing garlic, so he used to use old water-stuck cloves to clean his greenhouse, he would fervently swear that he killed mildew and any other pathogens, and obviously having been his grandfather who passed it on to his dad, his antibacterial powers were evidently quite well thought out.

Our modern high-tech world now has natural beaters, all but forgotten by nature, which are often absolutely harmless without chemicals being produced by any man to threaten the environment. Maybe we should look more closely at what our ancestors knew and seemed to forget.

How to Use It as Food and as a Health Remedy

Many people think the stinging nettle, Urticant dioic, is an irritating herb and generally seeks to eradicate it from the environment. However, you can make this delicious plant dishes and use it to boost your wellbeing.

The plant consists of a central root system, horizontalized and generally hidden stalks, which grow from the root and vertical stalks with their leaves and flowers from those horizontal stalks. The leaves lie in the young sprouts around the stalks all the way to the top. Finally, a top with many green flowers is grown around it. The root and horizontal stalks live for several years, and each spring, the vertical stalks grow.

You must harvest this plant as well as cook it just like a dish and use it in teas or extracts as a health remedy.

HOW TO GATHER As well as COOK NETTLE

Young stalks that emerge in the spring are the perfect material for this plant to use. You can still use the soft tops of older stalks, though, and then harvest the leaves if you catch the stalks and cut the leaves with a step upwards. For example, when you pick this herb, you will have on the palms.

You must then flush the material with water so that sand and soil are removed and cut into smaller pieces. You should then cook it like a potato. The water from the boiling cycle must not be spilled because it provides several valuable nutrients. Use it or drink it as a tea in your dishes. When boiled for a while, the plant no longer stings.

You could also dry the plant and store it as a tea or as a vegetable for later use. You could even press the juice out, or you can make nettle extracts.

Stinging nettle could also be used in soups as a very good degusting ingredient. In order to use it as a cure for illnesses, teas and extracts are also better made from it. You can use much more food material than you can eat as a portion of food by producing teas and extracts, thereby increasing the dosage of productive substances. You may also process the vertical stalks for this form of use.

FOUND THE NUTRIENTS in this plant

The nettle contains a lot of calcium and iron, and the herb contains more protein than most other plants. It contains a high amount of vitamin K when fresh, but this content decreases through drying.

There are also trace minerals in the nettle since they are not overexploited in infertile soils. For good health, most of these trace minerals were also necessary. The safety benefit of the plant is partially due to the high trace mineral content.

HOW STINGING NETTLE is good for the holy spirit.

Teas, Dishes, and extracts from this plant help to boost overall health and keep the body fresh. It has an especially strong rejuvenating effect on brain and skin functions. The rejuvenating impact on the skin is also seen after a few days when you take a decent amount of punching nettle each day.

Stinging nettle promotes proper functioning of the kidney and increases urine production. This is a safe treatment for hyperplasia of the prostate. Enhancing urinary output can improve water concentration and assist with cardiac and circulatory issues. The plant can also give nursing mothers better milk production.

The stinging of nettles counteracts inflammation and pain and can, therefore, be used for inflammatory diseases, such as rheumatism and allergies. A healthy treatment for respiratory problems such as sinusitis, rhinitis, hay fever, and asthma. It is ideal for calming irritated skin, and natural treatment for eczema and watery extracts of the herb can drink and rub on the skin for that purpose.

The plant may help cure anemia and other deficiencies in blood, partly because of the iron content. Since the high vitamin K content, juices, teas, and extracts from freshly grown plants are effective against bleeding. Remedies made from the dried plant lacked the silting effect on the skin. Rather, medicines made from dried plants are ideal for blood thinning.

HAVE YOU ANY HARMFUL EFFECTS?

There were no significant risks of stinging nettle. The rubbing feeling of the herb on the blank skin is clearly the side effect of stinging nettle. Contact with the fresh plant could also lead to eczema lasting several days.

Sticking nettle is often slightly annoying to the digestive tract, and vegetation or plant material may irritate the urinary bodies. Therefore, you should be careful more about the amount people use the plant when it starts to flower.

If you take blood thinners, take drugs for elevated blood pressure, or during breastfeeding, you should be careful when using the herb as a medicine.

## Mother Nature's Health Remedies

Americans learn basic school nutrition-four food groups, water, and vitamins. Yet emotional and spiritual sustenance was the essential food for human life missed.

Soul food (nutrition) tends to vary to some degree since some people really need and less of one thing, or something different together. Silence is one thing everyone wants. How much silence varies, of course, not only from person to person but at different times. Being outside with nature is one of the most efficient ways to meet your needs for silence.

Besides silence, people must be close to the four elements – Earth, water, air, and fire. Camping offers an ideal scenario where all four elements are integrated into one setting – campfire, the nearby stream, lake or river, and less polluted air in a rural setting.

Two blocks from a trailhead on the east side of the world 's largest municipal park-South Mountain-my home in Phoenix, AZ is a magical seven thousand areas stretching 17 miles west to east where I walk. Yes, campfires are approved and no water even during heavy rain; water stays for a while, but dirt, air, and plants are plentiful in low spots or creeks.

The Saguaro Cacti are the most abundant flowering vegetation and bear witness to the geological wonders. A broad, dense, fluted columnar stem of 18 to 24 cm in diameter with white flowers in spring, sometimes with many large branches (arms), which jut into the sky in its finest, most distinctive light-filled configuration. The roots of Saguaros are only 4-6 "deep that radiate as far as the plant is high. There is a deep root (taproot), reaching more than two miles into the earth.

The Saguaro is beautiful because it is beneficial. After the death of Saguaro, its wooden ribs can be used in the construction of roofs, fences, and furniture parts. Among the dead Saguaros are the holes that birds nestled on or "saguaro feet." Long before the cantina was made, Native Americans used this as water containers.

Saguaros grow exclusively in Arizona, New Mexico, and California in the Sonoran Desert. Water and temperature are the most important factors for development. If the temperature is too high, they can be destroyed by cold weather and frost. The Sonoran Desert has winter and summer rains, but during the rainy summer, the Saguaro retains its moisture to sustain itself in the dry season.

To which plants in your environment are you drawn? California Redwoods, Maple and Oak trees are among many favorites on the east coast of the country. In mid-October, the fall leaves are visible in brilliant orange, yellow, rust, and red beauty on an enormous pilgrimage through New England. But once a year, in fact, mind, body, and spirit are not properly protected.

Indoor water fountains and house plants are significant. Plants take carbon dioxide with water and sunlight, which produces photosynthesis and therefore releases glucose and oxygen. Rocks and shells are also useful for taking nature into your home setting. All of them contain a portion of the four elements.

Few people take the time to learn about the psyche and soul energy of nature. However, you will consider, if you investigate and pursue these ancient concepts, that nature itself holds the secret to an inner understanding of human existence and the role played by humans in the great Celestial Scheme.

The four components allow you to open up to the magic of creation. What do you hold in your home with the four elements? What opens you to life 's beauty? Who do you think is beautiful to remind you how life is wonderful to see?

Beauty is in the viewer's eye and whatever; it will nourish the mind and spirit. However, you must make aware that you are surrounded by the four elements and deal with them every day. Dashing or bathing counts with only hygiene and is no substitute for water in nature, as the highly toxic chemical is chlorine.

In addition, free antioxidant electrons fuel the earth. At light velocity, the electrons flow into your body as you touch the earth with bare feet or skin. When people are disconnected from either the natural negative load, we are more exposed to oxidation and inflammatory problems.

Research conducted by scientists and medical doctors who use all biological indicators, such as cortisol, cardiac bilirubin, cardiac variability, respiration, and white blood cell level, to assess if there is a difference between being grounded and not grounded reveals that all biological markers differ enormously when grounding (feet or bare skin that touches the ground directly 0).

Antiaging Foods for Health

The diet we eat starts with our healthy health intentions. Many people believe that swallowing a vitamin or exercise is all you need for good health. Homeostasis or balanced health is the result of many good things. But food, and much of it, is at its heart.

I have included a list of nutritious foods that facilitate healing. Such diets update the aging cycle, encourage weight loss, eradicate cancer and cardiovascular disease, and enhance healthy skin.

Learn how to choose and eat from the list below. A good meal would consist of a magnetic protein, vegetable (steamed or raw), and/or a few carbohydrates such as brown rice, beans, or even fruit.

"The inherent healing ability in each one of us is the greatest factor of our well-being. Our diet needs to be our medicine.

PRODUCE — These sections cover all vegetables. But the cruciferous vegetables such as broccoli, kale, spinach, roman lettuce, and brussels sprouts are especially essential. Know vegetables to cook. These are the most effective anti-aging foods that you can eat.

Green veggies contain beta carotenes and phytonutrients that are good therapies to prevent cancer, especially prostate, ovarian, and breast cancers.

Eating from the rainbow is just as necessary. Seek these basic foods in all forms and preparations. Fix salads and add veggies to your taste and spice. Start a routine of juicing or smoothie.

Here's a way I use. Steam your veggies-add a teaspoon of butter or olive oil and sprinkle with pepper and salt for 5 minutes. Add some grilled cheese. YUM, the trick here is to use SPICES that you want to try. I like tomatoes, artichokes, avocados, baby carrots and salads for raw veggies.

BERRIES – Blueberries contain an anthocyanidin nutrient. Whew!! Whew!! I can't even say it. These are very strong antioxidants that prevent cancer, macular degeneration, heart disease, and cancer. A curious fact is that there is resveratrol in red wine.

Resveratrol contains anti-aging anthocyanidins, which are known as a nutrient for heart and heart health. More anthocyanidins than red wine is present in blueberries. They are perfect in the morning or afternoon break with fruit salad, vegetable juice, or yogurt.

NUTS AND SEEDS — Nuts are usually healthy sources of nutrients, vitamin E, and good natural fats in our bodies. Almonds are better for heart health. Strong almonds, walnuts, pumpkin seeds, and sunflower seeds are my favorite combination. It's a perfect snack. Nuts also make a nice snack in the afternoon, and appetite stops on the streets.

FRUIT – Apples, grapes, kiwi, seeds, bananas, etc. The fruit is great anti-aging food. The fruit has significant quantities of fiber, which allows healthy absorption, contains antioxidants, and is a general purifier for the body.

A recent study has predicted that when everyone eats the five fruits and vegetables needed daily, we can decrease heart and cancer diseases by 50 —60%. For a break in the morning or afternoon, I like fruit in all different combinations.


LEAN PROTEIN – Eat small quantities of lean protein all day long. LEAN TURN ON THE METABOLIC ENGINE THAT BOURNS FAT THROUGHOUT YOUR Day even while you sleep.

Foods such as hormone-free chicken, turkey, eggs, lean beef cuts, beans, and fish can be a routine part of everyday diet. Fish have high DMAEs (like salmon) and promote skin health and texture.

Fish also carry high amounts of the overall health of vitamin D. One word of warning is to consider suppliers of heavy metal-free, steroid-free fish, and meats.


MUSHROOMS — Mushrooms help stop blood clotting from reducing blood vessel atherosclerosis. Mushrooms are a big source of manganese, potassium, phosphorous, selenium, copper, and zinc. These are also high in B3, B2, B6, B5, and iron vitamins.

We do have a number of phytonutrients available. In salads, soups, and stews, the mushrooms go well. Recommendations indicate that cooking time should not exceed 7 minutes.

BEANS and LEGUMES — Powerful mineral sources, especially molybdenum, manganese, phosphorus, magnesium, copper, potassium, and iron, are legumes and beans. They are also a high fiber source. For starters, 62 percent of the required day fiber is given by a cooked cup of pinto beans.

A total of 16000 people from many countries have been analyzed on the basis of their food intake. Their diet was monitored closely. The men who frequently ate beans and legumes reported an 82 percent decline in the risk of heart disease.

Some beans, such as pinto beans, have folate, which is a tremendous heart health nutrient. Bohemia is a very flavorful and good complex carbohydrate for sweet protein consumption.

GARLIC AND ONIONS — Sulphur compounds contain these allium veggies and give them strong scents. Research has shown that these veggies contain sulfur.

Prevent red blood cell anti-clotting, reduce LDL cholesterol, and elevated triglycerides. Garlic provides blood vessel lining protection and prevents blood coagulation causing a heart attack.

Dice first the onions, garlic or scallions and let them cook for a minimum of 5-10 minutes before mixing them. This activates the allium enzymes absolutely and optimizes their health-related properties. Add unbelievable flavor to your food, garlic, and onions. Use them strictly.

WATER — Most people do not see water in the balanced food profile of their people. Nevertheless, it is important. When we consider that our bodies represent 60-70% water, it must be a crucial factor in our health plan. Here are some interesting water facts:

- The main composition of our blood, tissues, and organs is water.
- Many nutrients pass through water through our bodies.
- Water is the key to removing toxins.
- Water is required for every purpose of the body.
- Water mills joints and acts as a shock absorber. Some arthritics may relieve pain by consuming water.
- Liquid water. Oil is a liquid. It dissolves nutrients and electrolytes and facilitates their diffusion through the body.
- Air regulates the temperature of the body. It keeps us moist when we're cold and cool when we're hot with sucking.

Do you know that the average American kept in his colons 7 to 25 pounds of fecal material? You will continue weight loss by increasing the intake of water. The colon is flushed with water.

The University of Loma Linda completed its research on 20,000 7th-day Adventists. We discovered that all people who drank at least five glasses of water a day were 50% less likely to die from heart attacks.

A further important point. The intake of coffee, soft drinks, fruit, and other beverages is not counted. Each person needs good quality water-filtered, not water bottled. Bottled water contains residues of plastic.

Body weight = 1 quarter/50 lbs. normal Optimum Intake

For, e.g., a person with 150 lbs. will require three-quarters of good quality water every day.

SOAP MAKING INSTRUCTIONS

---

### Soap Making Recipes

Handmade soap has many skin benefits, which tend to relieve conditions such as eczema, psoriasis, and acne. Soapmaking is now readily accessible on the Internet and in bookstores and involves hundreds of soap types. You will make your own natural soap items using only the ingredients that you choose to use in your soap until you've learned the fundamentals of soap production.

Foundation ingredients of soap recipe: lye (sodium hydrochloride) Purified water Fats and oil (lard, butter, olive oil, coconut oil) scent oils and essential oils the chosen soap recipe will include fats and oils of the correct type. Most soap producing recipes use animal fats, but vegetable shortening may also be used. Specific forms of oil are also used in soap recipes. Olive oil helps to moisturize the soap, while cocoa oil provides a strong lather effect on the soap. Other oils commonly used in recipes for soap preparation include almond oil, coconut oil, and sunflower oil. You must be careful to use the right mixture of fats and oils when making home-produced soap, because they have different "saponifying" properties, meaning, for example, you cannot substitute exactly the same quantity of lard with olive oil.

The ingredients that render soap formulas are scent oils and mineral oils. Fragrance oils do not appear to be used too commonly in beginning soap recipes because they contain soap and can interfere with the method of producing soap. On the other hand, essential oils are a little more costly but easy to use. Soap recipes typically state that you add fragrance oils in the trace stage, but the base oils may be used to incorporate essential oils faster. Fragrance and essential oils come in a wide variety of fragrances, and both have various aromatherapy and skin conditions. The types of natural ingredients are used in the soap recipes you see today: * Lavender soap recipes; lavender is an effective aromatherapy oil that is said to have a soothing effect. It is, therefore, soft on the skin and repellent insects.

* Simple, simple-sweet, chamomile recipes help alleviate tension and promote calm sleep.

* Citrus oil sap recipes; citrus, orange, and lime oils can give a calming fragrance to your soap and give it a soothing feeling.

Naturally, much of the aromatherapy and scent oils can be mixed to produce many more intriguing recipes. You will have a lot of fun experimenting with various aromas and combinations to produce your homemade soap with the right formula!

Marie Ackland-Soapmaking was a passion of mine, which gave me much pleasure and pleased me with the creation of a lovely scented soap bar from afar.

Instead, it was a full-time hobby for families and friends to love. Once a friend got up, I took it to a local art fair that I did and never looked back from that day. I now have a wonderful soap company that makes a decent profit and gives me much pleasure.

So, I love to teach soapmaking art 20 years on from my first set. It can be overwhelming at first, but if you know the basics and follow my techniques, you can still have fantastic soap.

Day soaps are extremely popular now that we are all searching for ways to save a buck. Since soap is homemade, there are no additives or other impurities in soap that are sold on the market. You can make soaps for your own use or give family and friends beautifully enjoyable presents. Homemade soaps are an easy and enjoyable weekend project.

Many of the recipes can be practiced very quickly, and the results are good creations. With colors and textures and tastes, you have several choices. The only thing you need to learn is a soap formula for your own shower. The method with all sorts of materials and procedures can be a bit daunting at first.

Fluid soap, vegetable soap, bath bombs, and several more are available. Liquid soap is now very popular because it doesn't leave a dry soap stain and needs the exfoliating benefits of loofah.

When dropped in the bathwater, bath bombs are a soap ball that makes the water soap and creates a bubble effect.

Vegetable soaps are a gentle soap that soothes your skin during your use. Palm soaps use a combination of oil-vegetable oil, shortening, cocoa butter, and lye.

Basic Soap Recipes From products you can find in your supermarket:

Recipe
• 30% olive oil
• 30% coconut oil
• 10% sunflower oils
• 5% sunflower oil

This recipe is just a tiny 6 bar pan, so I would have used 25 ounces of oil.
• Sunflower oil
• 5% sunflower oils


• 7.6 ounces. Olive Oil
• 7.6 ounces. Bacon
• 6.3 oz. Cocoon Oil
• 2.5 ounces. Sunflower Oil
• 1.3 ounces.
• 3.6 oz.
• 8 oz lye.
• 1.1 oz. of water.

Olive oil, Sunflower, and Lard oil will all be in the shop's daily cooking oil package. Castor oil is also used as a laxative in the pharmacy store. Coconut oil can also be paired with other food oils in the ethnic food market, or in larger markets.

If you have the method down, you have infinite possibilities to test what ingredients to add. Homemade soaps will power you and benefit those with allergic skin or allergies. You have the option to add ingredients that avoid an allergic reaction and soothe delicate skin. You cannot use fragrances, dyes, and other ingredients.

All of us need more than a book to learn how to produce soap. The basic method is harder to understand, and an amazing book and guide is available; that is what you need to talk about - it is a full tutorial that teaches you to step by step how to produce the soap you like.

## The Basic Soap Making Ingredients

Soap making is a complicated process, but soap-making materials are very simple: oils, lye, water, fragrances, dyes and other optional additives. The fats and oils in soap can be derived from vegetable or animal fat. Soaps derived from vegetable oils are usually smoother than those made from animal fat. Fixed oils-oils that can be heated to the high temperature without evaporation are the most important oils for soap production. Fixed oils contain a number of essential oils, including olive, palm and coconut oils.

There are two types of fats: saturated fats and unsaturated fats. Saturated fats make washing complicated.

These are typically firm in shape and must be melted before use; cacao and shea butters are excellent examples of saturated fat. Unlike other vegetable oils, unsaturated fats come in a liquid shape, and are also used to produce liquid soap. To make bar soap with these fats you have to blend with saturated fat, the tougher the bar would be.

Lye (also known as sodium hydroxide, potash, or caustic soda) has traditionally been hand-extracted from wood ashes. It is now available in many hardware and grocery stores. It is the component in which the oil or fats are hydrolyzed and converted into soap.

The salts and other contaminants in tap water make it less than ideal for producing soap. This is also safer to use fresh water, bottled water or spring water. Two types of fragrance oils exist: essential oils and fragrance oils. The scent oils are man-made and contain alcohol and are thus usually protected from drying up or damaging skin alcohol and other chemicals in the oil which can cause unexpected problems during the saponification process or totally destroy the soap mixture.

Essential oils are costlier and therefore easier to obtain, but a lower quantity is needed, usually just one or two drops, and since they are undiluted, they have a better fragrance. Until usage, study oils thoroughly; some may be unpleasant or even harmful to the skin. Different amounts are often needed for different oils, as some overwhelm others when equivalent quantity is used for both.

Avoid potpourri, candle scent oils and other solid, commercially manufactured fragrances as they frequently contain sharp, skin irritating chemicals. Whole or crushed herbs can be used, but in a first batch of soap they do not gain to their full ability. When you have herbs, the first thing to do is pick up the soap afterwards, and get the most of the herbs.

Colorants can be found in a shop for soap production.

There are also various natural ingredients to use in coloring soap, including ground clay, cocoa powder, tea, paprika, saffron and rattan jot. Avoid weaving cloth colors, hair dyes, candle dyes or soap paints; even though they are labelled as "non-toxic," they are not healthy for a long time to come in contact with the skin, so they can stain the skin.

There are places where crayons can be applied to coloration soap, so long as they are manufactured from stearic acid (most crayons are manufactured now), although there is some debate in this field.

The resulting soap will be contaminated based on the oils used in the process.

Various preservatives, such as vitamins E, C, and A, can also be used, and are safe for the health. These vitamins are present in various oils. To exfoliate, sand or pumice should be added to the soap. Few metals such as platinum, copper, nickel, or aluminum can also be applied to make the light soap white for antibacterial properties.



The use of an immersion blender to produce handmade soap accelerates the process of saponification and saves lots of time. In addition to reducing trace time, isolation issues in the soap should be reduced. ATTENTION! You can have frozen chunks of milk to mix when you make goat milk soap. Should not put your dip blender on some frozen bits. You could snap the blade and permanently destroy your blender.

The finest mixers are not necessarily the most expensive. You don't need many fancy soap-making machines. Anything functional, strong, reliable, easy to clean, and the store is required. Choose the one that best suits your wants, conveniences, and desires. You will find the right mixer for all your recipes! With the right soap supplies, you can save time, effort, and money in the long run! Thousands of bolts are available on the market. What do you know which mixer is the best for you? Let's look at other aspects and find the right mixer for you.

WEIGHT: What's the mixer heavy? You may want a lightweight blender if you're in the soap making market. For the year-round preparation of huge quantities of goat milk oil. It would be easy to operate with a heavy blender, but if you use it regularly, it might become tiresome.

POWER: These bolt blenders are approximately.25 hp (hp) with a total output of 200 watts. Basic mixers have average horsepower range from.40 to.80 with a power of 300 to 600 watts. The fastest blenders are up to roughly 2.0 hp with a power of 1500 watts.

Once combined, soap produces a smoother feel. You will need a powerful engine immersion blender, but it does not have to be the most powerful in the industry. You must learn how to use the mixer to make homemade soap. Sporadically using it. When you keep pouring soap constantly, you would more than certainly flame out the engine! When this happens, you are going to stir with a spoon, yes, for several hours.

Battery-operated blenders do not seem to be very long powered. They can be used, but you must have to keep them filled to have the ability to blend your soap.

Pick: Look at the blender's edge. Is he made of stainless steel, or is he made of plastic? Some argue that the blade in stainless steel is much stronger than the rubber. When using hard plastic blades, they can crack, tear, crumble, or even melt. Could the razor be removed? Is cleaning easy? Will it be quickly replaced?

BLENDING: Is the blender easy or difficult to handle? Some may claim that the suction force of blenders is too strong to lose control and management. Never immerse the motor (handheld portion) of the water or liquid immersion blender! This portion of the mixer is never dirty. Only submerge it, not further than the wall length.

POWER CORD: How long longer does the power cord last? Could it be retracted? For a long power cable, you can switch through your kitchen or anywhere you blend. With a retractable cord, it's convenient to clean and pack. For handmade soap, you don't have to have a long or retractable power cable. They are convenient. They're easy.

SIZE & COMFORT: Does your hand suit well? Is it too big or too short to tie your hand? Is it too slippery? Is it easy to position the controls? Most bolts suit the hand proportionally, but because you are the one to use it, it is important in terms of size and comfort.

SPEEDS: Many blenders have only one velocity, some variable velocity. So long, so you blend the soap for an appropriate period of time, making sure all the ingredients are properly combined, it doesn't really matter the difference in rpm. Faster speeds will reduce some mixing time. This is only easy to have different speeds.

CLEAN-UP: How easy is your immersion blender to clean? Are the blade and/or shaft reusable to clean up easily? Are the dishwasher blade and/or shaft safe? Another easy way to clean your blender is first to toggle it on or unplug it and then drain the excess soap, immerse it in hot soapy water, toggle it on again and then continue mixing as usual. This allows the blade, shaft, and under the guard to be swept. You should also shut the blender off and run the blade and the shaft mild or hot tap water to rinse it in the tub. Care should be taken to remove water from electronic controls and the engine. Never bring a blender into a dishwasher, but just a free, removable portion of the dishwasher!

COLORS: Stick blenders, green, purple, black, gray, brushed chrome, etc. come with a variety of colors. Black and rubbed chromium do not reveal stains as light colors. It's just your pick.

SHAFT: Is the shaft silver or plastic? Many claims that the chrome shaft is much more washed than the rubber, leading to stains.

NOISE: Is working quietly? Loud, noisy blenders can be annoying for some people, particularly if regularly used.

STORAGE: Most mixers are fitted with a storage frame. You can install the immersion blender near, comfortably, in a cupboard or storage unit, or lock it inside, along with its other accessories.

EXTRAS: Many blenders have additional accessories: whisk, beaker, blade, and safer: keep your hands still away from blade(s) when used. Switch the blender off or unplug if it's not in service.

READ Comments: Read any consumer feedback before settling on the right blender for you. You will read lots of user feedback (immersion), strong or low star scores on Amazon.com. Most people will read consumer comments online.

RETURN RULES: As with any commodity, before buying, search for return or swap rules. Save all receipts. Delete all receipts.

WARRANTY: Test the warranty much like any good you purchase.


Glycerin Soap Making Instruction - Problem Solving

Most of the issues with the Melt & Pour Soap are due to the soap base temperature. Using the botanicals, oils, and embedding at the right moment will make an outstanding soap.

When the temperature is right, very little can go wrong. Glycerin soap is extremely versatile. If you don't like the look, melt it down again and continue again.

Many typical issues and what to do to solve them are described below.

The soap was overheated, losing humidity, or dropped in the fridge. Add 5% glycerin and melt again.

Melting is hidden soap. Soap temperature over embedded objects was too hot or soap too thin. Try to ice the embedding soap and mist with alcohol.

Soap slipping and falling out of the bar inserted. The base of the soap is too dry. Until embedding, let the soap cool. Spritz the alcohol sections before bonding.

The bar finished is slimy and sticky. You didn't tie the soap. You didn't. Glycerin retains moisture in the soap. Remove it and tie it.

Soap coated separates. Separates. Spritz all sections of alcohol, but then pour the 2nd layer on only as the first one is ready to take the second one into weight.

And tastes terrible and has been overheated, which causes it to smoke. Adding scent won't help.

Colors are bleeding. Bleeding. You used the wrong coloring form. Do not use food coloring, it will rust, spill into other colors, and you will dye the skin if you have used too many.

The soap is not translucent anymore. You may overheat the soap or have applied a clarity-changing additive. Honey, beeswax, or oats, for example.

Soap does not lather. Soap does not lather. You have exceeded the amount of oils indicated in your soap. Extra oil coats and causes the bubbles to burst under their weight. The oil bubbles to the rim in serious situations, giving the soap an oily appearance.

Botanical goods are brown. For botanicals, it is not uncommon to change color. Even flowers dried by air for months can change color and become moldy if kept in the soap for longer periods.

Floating and exfoliating botanicals sink. That is another concern with temperature. The soap should be cool enough to form a surface and to touch the bottle warmly. When the viscosity is right, it is possible to add botanicals and exfoliants. Mind that the soap will float or sink.

The soap is not translucent anymore. You may overheat the soap or have applied a clarity- additive. Honey, beeswax, or oats, for example.

Soap does not lather. Soap does not lather. You have surpassed the amount of oils indicated in your soap. Extra oil coats and causes the bubbles to burst under their weight. The oil bubbles to the rim in serious situations, giving the soap an oily appearance.

Some of the best suggestions I've had come from my students, and we do it in three hours. Have a look. Have a go. It's simple, quick, and so imaginative you can be.



### Seven Secrets to Choosing A Safe, Healthy Pet Food

Do you choose dry food or canned food? What brand?  So many different brands exist, all forms and sizes of pet food are available, and pet owners have very little information to base their decisions on (other than advertising). Okay, depending on your information about the pet food industry, tighten your seatbelt, this could be a bumpy journey! You're about to understand seven secrets of pet food-well kept secrets. Sit back, brace yourself, and continue to read.

Science Diet, 'promises' precisely balanced food through continuous research and high-quality food with the support of your Vets and sells only for a 20 lbs. bag for about $21.00. Then there are numerous animal foods that sell for $30.00 or more for a bag of 20 lb. "Premium Dog Food," Highest Quality. Then the same happens to cat owners... do you want Whiskas, who says that 'all we do is make cats happy! Or do you choose one of the high-end cat foods that claim to be a healthy, happy cat, but cost three times more?

Now, there are issues with the pet food alert owners like 'Has this food been remembered? 'or' is it the next food to be remembered? '...' Is my animal safe?' 'It's confusing, Wow! And frightening too! What exactly should an animal owner do? How about a few things to discover! It's not that overwhelming, armed with the experience of certain mysteries of pet food.

# 1 Secret ...

Most meat feeds use common terms such as options and prices, but only a few use qualities or chosen food products. The 'secret' means that pet foods cannot make any claims or references on their label or advertising about the quality or grade of their ingredients according to the rules of the pet food industry. You see, the word 'premium' does not mean that the food ingredients are premium when they relate to pet food. In pet foods, premium neither describes the product (cannot) nor describes the product consistency (cannot). It's a marketing term, and that's everything. In compliance with the pet food industry's own rules and regulations, "There is no relation to the standard or value of the product" (regulation PF5 d 3). Words such as premium, choice, or quality are simply marketing or sales terms. The terms describing the quality of the food should not be interpreted.

Then why is it not appropriate for a pet food company to tell the consumer the consistency of the ingredients? Isn't an animal owner worth knowing what they're buying? This brings me to the next secret ...

Code number 2 ...

When I can compare "people's food" to pet food for a second, we all know that people's foods have different qualities. There's White Castle, and there's Outback Steak House (anyone else's favorite) (I'm sorry, I love the little guys!). Meat and potatoes are served in all restaurants. You will have a few hamburgers as well as an order of fries in White Castle for under $3.00. You will get a steak as well as a baked potato for around $16.00 at the Outback. Both beef and potatoes are consumed – but you do know that there are major dietary variations between a fast-food hamburger and a steak.

The challenge with the pet food business is that most animal owners do not believe in pet food in the same way. They don't think that there are fast food types of pet foods, and more nutritious pet foods are available at restaurants. In fact, a young man experimented with his own diet some years ago-eating only fast food for 30 days. Three meals a day, he had a great deal of weight, blood pressure, and cholesterol in just one month of fast food. Now, imagine that your cat would eat that kind of food all his life.

Well then back to our two foods, both would analyze with a percentage of protein, carbohydrates, and fat if your food in White Castle were compared with a chemical analysis of your food in Outback. No matter whether you find an Outback steak a better protein content than a sandwich - it will also be evaluated as a meal. The analysis does not measure protein quality.

So here is the key. All pet foods are supplied with a guaranteed report showing the protein, sugar, fiber, and moisture content of the food. The True answer lies in the content of protein, fat, and so on percentages.

Chicken feet can be analyzed as a protein in a chemical examination of a pet product since they have very little nutrients. And indeed, a cow euthanized by a disease that made it unfit for human use will be treated as a protein, but it could be considered unsafe for eating. It could be considered harmful. The ingredients of both-chicken feet and the euthanized cow-are permissible and are commonly used in pet food. You see, the secret in the animal food industry is that producers get their ingredients from a WIDE-OPEN door. The only strict rule they have to follow is for an adult dog food to analyze with 18% protein and for an adult cat food to analyze 26% protein. The origins for possessing such quantities range from "human-class" foods to chicken paws, euthanized animals, plant proteins, and even man-made artificial proteins.

Animal feed labels do not have to indicate the sources they are using to obtain 18 percent or 26 percent protein. To make matters worse... Quality manufacturers - those companies which use 100% ingredients of human-grade - cannot tell customers or potential customers that their products are ingredients of quality and human-grade.

Then how do you know whether the food of your pet uses chicken feet or euthanized cows?

# 3 Secret ...

If the terms luxury and preference literally mean little with respect to pet food consistency and if pet foods use chicken feet and euthanized animals in their diets, how does a pet owner know what their pets' food is?

This great mystery is hidden in the meanings of ingredients. In comparison to foods for 'men,' where the food should be looked at to determine its consistency, pet food is somewhat special. Each 'people' food must conform with strict USDA (Agriculture Department of the United States) and FDA guidelines. The same does not apply to pet food. Chicken feet and euthanized cows, for obvious reasons, are not allowed in people to eat-they have no nutritional value, or they can be hazardous to consume. The same does NOT apply to pet food. The only way you can tell if your pet's diet is made up of these chicken feet or euthanized cows is to ask what recipes they use.

The 'meat and bone meal' traditional pet food ingredient is a blend of several different leftover ingredients from the human food market. The 'meat and bone feed' components could include anything from cow's heads, bellies and intestines, to (horrific but true) euthanized animals such as veterinary office cows, horses and dogs, and cats, animal shelters and farms. The pet food contains the drug pentobarbital used to euthanize the animal, alongside those euthanized animals. Meat and bone meal can also include left-wing restaurant fat, and diseased (including cancerous) meat tissue cut off from animals slaughtered. In other words, this commonly used ingredient is a mixture of the human food industry's highly inferior and potentially dangerous links.

The 'meat by-product' or 'meat by-product meal' ingredient in pet food is pretty much the same as 'meat and bone meal.' It is a very weak product for pet food that actually includes who knows what.

'Animal Digest' is another similar ingredient.

As far as chicken feet I have mentioned above are concerned, this item can be found in the 'Chicken By-Product' or 'Chicken By-Product food' or 'Poultry By-Product Food' ingredients. The leftover of the chicken or poultry division-including, but not limited to, chicken feet, skin, and intestines, including certain feathers, chicken, or poultry heads. The health of the bird does not matter – ill, well, killed, dying ... all these ingredients are used.

So, here's what you need to do ... Before you buy any pet food, toss the bag over, and look at the ingredients list carefully. The above ingredients are mentioned in the first 5 or 10 ingredients. If you see any of these ingredients, it's my suggestion not to buy it. Remember-the the euthanized animals and chicken feet analyze as protein. This is all that is needed in pet food-just the right analysis.

Some pet food manufacturers use grains and chemical additives to improve the percentage of protein in grain products in this category. That is precisely the cause of the recall in March 2007 of pet food-chemical proteins. In addition to a grain drug (Wheat Gluten, Corn Gluten, or Rice Gluten), two separate chemical compounds that have NO nutritional benefit in pets yet were tested as protein have been introduced to have a cheap protein only. Thousands of animals died, and many more became sick because the mixture of these two compounds would induce urinary and kidney blockage. Again, their trick is that the food needs to be tested as having a certain protein content-no one has to supply a standard meat protein.

As regards the ingredient listing-you need to take note of the number of cereals (wheat, corn, rice) and/or the amount of grain products (corn gluten, whole maize, ground maize, whole wheat, wheat gluten, ground wheat, brown rice, rice, brawer rice, soy and on) in each of the first five ingredients. If you find more than one grain in the first five ingredients-this means that this animal feed acquires some of its protein from the grains.

Why is it important to know why protein obtained from grains? Several factors-research first show that both cats and dogs need a meat meal and survive on it. If pet food produces protein from grain sources, the pet does not get the meat it needs to grow. Secondly, if the grain products are maize gluten, wheat gluten, or rice gluten, you fear chemicals such as melamine, which are used specifically to promote protein processing. Melamine, by the way, is one of the chemicals suspected to be the cause of the pet food recall in March 2007. And with grains, there's another concern-aflatoxin. Aflatoxin is a lethal mold native to maize, wheat, and soy, and blamed for many other pet food reminiscences that you actually never heard about. Diamond Pet Food in December 2005 included moldy grains which killed more than 100 animals before the product was recalled – all due to aflatoxin.

I recommend that any pet food containing maize, wheat, or soy be avoided in any variation. The chance is just too high.

Do You Choose Dry Food or Canned Food?

# 4 Trade ...

I have more ideas to search for in the lists of additives ... natural preservatives. The use of chemical preservatives is a well-kept secret for the pet food industry. BHA / BHT are very popular chemicals used in pet foods and have been linked to tumors and cancer by science. Another popular preservative is ethoxyquin with documented cancer risks. Ethoxyquin is allowed ONLY in human foods due to its very small proportions in some spices. However, pet food is allowed to a much greater extent.

You will look for BHA / BHT and ethoxyquin, listed somewhere if you check the ingredient lists. BHA / BHT is widely used to retain the fat in the product that is usually mentioned above. Search for any of these chemicals at the end of the list of ingredients. I wouldn't personally touch pet food containing this chemical preservative. You want a natural pet food - 'natural mixt tocopherols' or 'vitamin E' are popular natural preservatives.


# 5 Secret ...

The right food for the pet is very well-made food that uses ingredients of a high standard. How do you discover that? This must be simple enough. You already understand that pet food manufacturers can't make any statement about the quality or quality of ingredients, but only to contact the manufacturer to find out the quality or quality of your pet food.

So, tell, contact the company and ask: Is your Quality Dog Food and Quality Cat Food made with human-grade ingredients? It may be that you obtain the answer: yes, we use human-grade ingredients – if only a few ingredients are human grade. Here's the trick to ask ... ask if they are certified as APHIS European.

The APHIS European accredited animal feed producers promise that the products in their pet food are of high quality. APHIS-Services for Animal Plant Health Inspection-is a USDA division. APHIS European certification offers this pet food manufacturer the chance to ship their food/treatments to Europe. European countries require all ingredients to be human grades when importing pet food from the USA, which requires this certification. The majority of pet food producers with European certification APHIS don't export their goods to Europe – they use it as a way of showing their customers the better quality of their ingredients.

Again, you're not going to see this on the label — it is not permitted. You have to call and ask the manufacturer. Often times, when you ask about APHIS certification, the pet food representative does not know what you are talking about, if so, you could even assume they weren't

APHIS European certified. European APHIS certification is a reward for pet owners-any pet food manufacturer is not required or suggested to take the extra steps to achieve it. Some pet foods make a special effort to tell their customers they really care about the quality of their products. Personally, I wouldn't order pet food, which doesn't.

And by the way, if you can't even reach the pet food manufacturer, or you can't make a quick call back in time, lose your number! Any company which does not prioritize customer questions-is not worth your business!

# 6 Secret ...

Minerals are required in human diets and in our pets' diets. Iron, Copper, and zinc are popular in pet foods. Just as they are-copper, iron and zinc are rocks, which are very difficult to use for anyone or pet. Science has developed different ways to absorb minerals (human and pet) into the body to enhance absorption and help the organism even more. This experimental discovery has been called chelating or protein enhanced for years. Minerals are absorbed approximately 60% better than minerals alone by the chelating or protecting process.

This secret detects the minerals that are chelated or proteins in your pet diet. Please remember the minerals on the packaging of your pet food, below the ingredients page. You are looking for minerals read 'cotton' or 'chelated copper.' If you just see the minerals on the list, your pet is like Halloween's Charlie Brown saying, 'I've got a rock.' If you are looking for the best, chelated, or proteinate minerals for your pet is one of the best foods!

Secret # 7 Secret ...

This secret is referred to as 'friendly bacteria.' Though 'friendly bacteria' sounds somewhat frightening, the reason lies in the intestinal system of your animals. A large part of the immune system of your animals can be found in the intestinal system. Maintaining a healthy immune system helps to keep the animal healthy. This friendly bacterium is similar to that found in yogurt, but it is introduced in pet food in a way to prevent it from being destroyed by the cooking process.

Your seven secrets help you find your four-legged friend's absolute healthiest and best pet food. Armed with these secrets – now you know how to find the best food you can for your pet! An animal feed that can extend its life and avoid early aging and disease. I urge you to subscribe to my monthly magazine Petsumer Report (TM), if you don't want to bother doing the homework involved. I do all my homework for you through Petsumer Report (TM)-every month, I review and rate over 40 different pet food, toys, and pet supplies. This is the ONLY publication of its kind, which gives animal owners the information that is needed about pet products.

I just want to share a few more things ...
Two meals a day are the safest way to feed the adult dog or cat. The food they eat with two meals is better used than only one meal per day. If you are feeding your animal one meal a day, divide the same amount into two meals, and feed in AM and PM.

You should be aware that all canned and moist pet foods have moisture ranging from 70% to 85% anywhere. This means 70 to 85% of food can or pouch is useless nutrition – its water. Our pets need water, especially cats, don't have enough water to drink. However, because all canned or humid foods are mainly water, they are not nutritional enough to be fed a strictly canned or moist diet. Use a canned as well as moist product to add to your pet's diet – not just as food.

The better pet foods are genetically conserved (secret # 4)-but the pet foods are natural ... freshness. Notify you of the expiration date on your product label for dogs-usually in dry pet products that have been naturally processed (not so many moist products due to cannery-very little recycling needs) the expiration date is about one year and 18 months from the date of its manufacture.

If you intend to adjust the diet of your dogs, please contact your veterinarian first. The improvements you make to your pet will also be told by your veterinarian. Do not even take chances. Don't take chances. And if you turn pet food, slowly change it. I always recommend 1/4 new food to the pet owners for 4-7 days, 1/2 to 1/2 for an additional 4-7 days, and so on. Food switching can cause intestinal disorder quickly! It's short term, but we don't want bowel disorder!!!

Finally, because you already know that dogs and cats have a much better sense of smell than people. Your food bowl can be a rich smell – good and bad alike. Sometimes an animal refuses to eat just because it smells a previous food in its bowl. Plastic food and bowls of water retain the worst smell. And stainless-steel bowls are surprisingly like that. A ceramic bowl is the best type of food, as well as a water bowl. They retain the least smell.

## Pet Preparation Prior to Disaster Striking

June arrives rapidly, and for most coastal areas, the fear of a storm is creeping into our heads.

The safety of our homes, pets, and ourselves worry us.

Hurricanes are not the only threats that our health and that of our animals will face. The list of events that could happen is made up of hurricanes, disasters, tornadoes, protests, and terrorist attacks.

It's important to have a plan. Hurricane Katrina was a disaster that not only displaced thousands of people but also displaced many animals, and sadly many were also killed. It is said that about 44% of the victims of Hurricane Katrina were livestock owners who would not abandon their livestock.

Until Katrina hit our country in the face of disasters was not too pet friendly. Most, if not all, did not allow animals of any type to be taken to a designated shelter.

Many states currently provide owners and the pets with shelters provided they comply with certain restrictions. However, Red Cross shelters do not require dogs. It is not their rule, and it is the rule of local health services. A Red Cross shelter is for those who have no animals, fear animals, or have allergies to animals.

It is up to "you" the animal owner to search the grounds to see the shelters have animals and what size and type of animal are permitted.

You and your pet must be at the top of your list of things to do in the future. The problem with advance preparation is that many of our people go in the "denial-mode." We tell ourselves that, regardless of what the disaster is, "it won't involve us."

So what is a pet owner supposed to do? I will give you some tips in the following paragraphs about how to keep the cat or dog as safe as humanely as possible. The important thing is to know that you have to prepare for a disaster.

A catastrophe kit must be large enough to contain everything your pet normally needs for at least seven days. It should be washable (a tightly-fitting plastic container) and labeled "cat or dog in case of disaster."

• Food: Pack your pet 's brand for cooking, both dry and frozen. Smaller cans are better because pets eat less in a disrupted environment.

Take a can opener (although sometimes they do not work even if the cans have lift tabs).

Food bowls and plastic lid cover for unsaturated canned food. Keep open cans in a cooler unconsumed. A spoon or two can help to prepare the canned food.

• Air: Nearly a week of drinking. Do not keep water for longer than three months at a time in an emergency package and store it coolly in the dark.

A water bowl with a small container of bleach to be used to purify undrinkable water, if necessary.

• Hygienic supplies: kitty litter and cat litter pan. Take enough litter to use with small plastic bags for at least a week to clear the litter when cleaning out the box.

Take a "pooper scooper" as well as plastic sacks for your dog to dispose of the waste.

• Washing materials: Incident paper towels for a washing litter box, food bowls, cage, or container. Cleaning materials.

Dish soap and other dry-cleaning disinfectants for containers, carriers, and other quantities.

• Pictures: Have recent photos of the pet, or if you have to make posters if your pet gets lost, take several photos or make copies.

Get a photo of your cat, perfect for distinguishing whether the cat is missing, and someone finds it. This is extremely important.


• Veterinary Information: Recent records of shots and vaccinations of your pet will be required.

You must take any medicines your animal is currently taking.

Write on a piece of paper the name, address, and telephone number of Vet. Additionally, include a note authorizing someone other than you to receive emergency treatment for the pet if you are not available.

Also, have your name, all the phone numbers available to you, addresses, and other info so you and your animal can be found separately.

Put all of this information in a plastic zip-lock bag.


• Collars, tags, and ID: make sure your cat wears a ruptured collar with an ID tag.

Have your dog always wear one.

Get a microchip for your pet and register with the national registry.

Have multiple ID tags if you lose.

Use your cat's harness to keep it on a leash, do not rely on the neck. Many cats with collars were missing because they could break rid of them. Have the cat practice at home with a harness for a couple of hours,

Get many leashes (one can get lost) and keep the animals on a leash if they are not in a cage or carrier.

Know at all times where your pet is.


• Various items: toys, towels, dry shampoo, flea protection, and treatments.

• Crate or carrier: Make sure the cake or carrier is large enough for the pet to move around comfortably, and if necessary, there will be room for food and water.

Crates (for dogs) take up lots of space, and the ideal product would be a collapsible cable with a robust lock.

A small and medium-sized dog might possibly contain a collapsible workout pen, just make sure that the dog can't dig out or crawl under it. Close it with a pin driven to the ground and attached to the plumb.

• Place a small kit of first aid that contains antiseptic wipes, gauze, bandages, a medical cream recommended by your veterinarian, several tweezers and scissors, and a cold/hot package.

Hold in a tub that is waterproof.

These are just a few suggestions to help you prepare for a catastrophe. The most important thing is to be ready to move when the time comes.

If you wonder whether or not your pet will be taken, ask yourself this question, "Should I leave a young child here to cope?"

What can you do if you can't take your pet?

With you? This is the case with a hurricane or inundation. Do not leave your pet in case of a fire or a tornado warning.

Do not leave your cat outside if you face a storm. A bathroom, wardrobe, or room without too many windows is a good starting point. Keep the pet there if you have a cellar.

Here's where a "self-feeder" comes in handy for dried milk. Load it with as much dried food as it is going to bear. If you have many creatures, get several feeders. If it is not possible to feed yourself, leave dried food in bins that can touch dogs or cats. Leave plenty of water in unlockable containers.

Leave a couple of clothes you recently wear with your cat, and your scent will provide warmth.

Wait for a mess when you go home.

Placed all the details on the pet's ID tags.

Leave the name and information of your Vet together with a note authorizing someone else than you to receive treatment for your pet if necessary. Put it in a plastic bag and nail it to a wall or a door so that it is visible.

If there is a risk of a flood, you must provide the pet with higher elevations.

The cellar is definitely not the place to keep your pet in the event of a flood. If you have an idea of the potential flood level, build some kind of area to allow the animal to climb to stay dry. Pile up furniture and create a space for the pet to reach. Make sure your pet has water and food available for eating on the floors and in the higher areas.

Don't tie your dog or chain it up if you leave the dog outside. Dogs may be left in the garages, barns, cockroaches, or even on a flat roof. If you are sunny, provide a big board, since a roof can be very hot and pet pads can be burnt.

Whenever you walk your house, make sure that it can be higher and that your pet can eat and drink food and water.

Do not leave your pet with medications, vitamins, or supplements; just have dry food and drink.

If your pet is a mouse, you will obey the same directions. Making sure that the cat has a place to escape in case of high water and that food and drink are stored there.

Refrigerators, high entertainment centers, or a shelf in a closet can ensure your cat 's safety. Keep a litter box in the location you've selected for cats.

Making arrangements with a neighbor to keep an eye on your pet when the disaster doesn't happen is a good idea. Offer your neighbor if you are not available, the requisite veterinarian details, and a notice to permit care.

Above all, be prepared and prepared.

When you go on vacation, please check whether your animals have a disaster plan with the kennel or the person who cares for them. This is where it is important to plan on your part. Ready your disaster kit to be used if necessary.

Leaving a pet is a very nervous thing to do, and don't do it if it isn't the only thing you can do. Just writing which sentence will have reduced me to tears, because I know that under no circumstances could I leave my pets.

If necessary, however, please do your best to ensure your pet's safety and well-being.

Disasters arise, and you should be prepared for them.

## HEALTH POSITIVE IMPLICATIONS

### Understanding Holistic Health

Many people are looking for a more holistic approach to health today in order to meet their health needs, but don't understand what it means or how it will benefit them. Consumers are increasingly aware that our current health care system has more than one failure, and action is necessary, but are afraid or distracted by other's negative perceptions and natural health skepticism based on misinformation and lack of understanding.

Most skepticism about alternative health methods is motivated by the unfortunate fact that modern medicine is trying to discredit alternative healing methods, because operations and pharmaceuticals are much more profitable for them, not for real reasons. The issue of alternative health always raises the question of Thomas, who shouts quackery and voodoo. You can learn that without a result, they have attempted a therapeutic approach or that they have an odd side effect or even feel worse.

Here are a few important things to consider. Their experience may be valid, but this does not mean that it is valid for all, and certain factors that lead to their experience may exist. We can very easily find another group of people who have had great success and have no side effects with exactly the same therapy.

Because not everyone's body responds in exactly the same way to a particular treatment or healing approach, even if you have the same disorder with another human, each of you has individual body chemistry and physiology, and the same illness will have an entirely different mechanism or effect. Each of these factors has an influence on the results. In fact, someone with a kidney, lymph system, endocrine system, or other dysfunctional organ or system may have a very different response than someone who has healthy organs and systems.

Just because one approach to treatment is ineffective for one person, it will not work for you or others, and this does not mean that "all" holistic care is ineffective. Results can be entirely different from individuals. It takes several trials and errors to figure out what fits well for your biochemistry in other conditions.

Therefore, if we speak of a holistic wellness approach or conventional prescription products, that is real. If we talk about natural therapies or prescription medications, what is good for one does not work for another, but the overall holistic wellbeing is much better and much more stable. Hundreds of thousands of people are dealing with serious side-effects, getting worse, having more severe health problems, or even dying from prescription drugs. These events, on the other hand, are rare in the field of natural health.

In reality, holistic health or natural health was far longer than traditional or "new" medicine. Plants and medicines have widely been used for millennia by many cultures, and most prescription medications find their origins in herbal medicine. The common and popular aspirin, for example, came from an herb called white willow bark.

Nevertheless, it is necessary for others to be unaware that it does not necessarily mean that if anything is normal, it should be free of side effects, problems, or dangers. Most doctors themselves have a clear knowledge of the process they use before they do their research.

Herbs, plants, vitamins, minerals, or any alternative treatment method can be as powerful as a prescription and requires a great deal of training and research to ensure the desired results are reached. They should be taken or carried out by an experienced health care provider as prescribed. For example, some holistic treatments that work for depression can have a negative impact on someone with Parkinson's.

Ineffective can be too much or too little of a specific herb, but too much of a vitamin or mineral is just as bad as insufficient. Even in natural substances, there can be complications or interactions, as a herb or even treatment method such as massage or acupuncture can counteract and revive another approach to treatments, and vitamins and minerals work together.

Furthermore, herbs and other natural substances can interact with prescription drugs and reduce their efficacy and vice versa. It is very important for you to consult a complete healthcare provider and disclose all medicines and conditions before taking medicine.

The quality of the product or service that you use is another important issue that can have an impact on the results of a holistic health solution. It is also vital for you to do your homework in this area and only use reputable companies' products and services. The area of natural health is not immune to fraud and scams. You need to be a diligent and informed consumer irrespective of your path.

Freeing ourselves from the old way of thinking that conditions us to believe that medication and surgery are the best way of treatment can be fearsome and difficult. At first, it may seem alien, threatening, or strange, but you can see that it makes a lot of sense when you get the facts about health.

Holistic health offers us a wealth of wholesome approaches from the treatment of herbal medicines and nutritional supplements to massages. It offers us acupuncture, yoga, detoxification, lifestyle changes, the environment, diet and the cleaning of the column, and chiropractic manipulation, meditation.

The patient works with the health provider as a team, and is encouraged to participate actively in the health plan, learn about their condition and participate in a variety of self-care techniques and practices.

In contrast to modern medicine, which tries only to suppress symptoms, holistic medicine seeks to correct the health condition whilst also finding the underlying cause. Instead of putting everybody on a cookie-cutter plan, holistic health care is a complete approach that is tailored to the specific needs of every person.

The ultimate goal is to allow each person to achieve the highest level of wellbeing, to work and to live as completely as possible regardless of the existence and absence of illness.

## Health Care - The Middle-Class Nightmare

Say you 're a normal middle-class Joe. Wait, you don't most have to because you're one. That's why you're going to hear what I have to say here. It's hard to keep your jobs, to cover new and rising taxes, to pay your bills on time and to keep struggling against the continuously inflating health care costs.

To survive in the current economy, businesses must take steps to reduce costs in any way they can. Sadly, this means layoffs, plant closings, and benefits for many of us. Those applying for new jobs are also expected to opt for an expensive health care plan. In the end, they are expected to pay extra for existing health care policies that have less coverage or no longer have any support at their fingertips. The question you have to ask yourself here is:

How much do I need health insurance?

Take a little time and return to last year's medical bills. I believe over 80 percent of you have spent at least almost as much on the health care premiums as you did on real medical bills. Tell yourself again, then. So badly do I like health insurance?

Around this point, I like to mention that I know that everyone's special circumstances and that for certain reasons, certain people are left with what they have. The following are some thoughts I had about comparing survival shopping:

1. Many patients visit a specialist 2-3 times a year and may have one routine prescription. They are the people I spoke to earlier in this 80 percent. If you are one of those people, a health plan with a higher deductible and a co-payment is a good way to save some money. More pocket spending is available, but lower premiums are available, and coverage is still available in the case of a serious illness or injury. Insurance firms make much of their profits from the citizens in this 80 percent community, and they have office buildings about the size in Rhode Island. By contrasting what you have now, you can save money to help cover your bills or consider a package that is affordable because you don't have one at all.

Don't believe that what you have to choose from is what your boss offers you for options. Since the industry has reduced ratios and new policies providing fewer coverage, health care packages are not what they used to be. Hundreds of businesses are on the Internet searching for your company urgently. Take the time to compare. And if you don't get 80 percent, what's the benefit that takes a few minutes to get some free quotes? Maybe you're happily shocked. Once, I know there are different circumstances with different individuals. And you have to do what is more important to you.

2. Another way to save money is to purchase your online pharmacy drugs. This is especially beneficial for those who cannot afford medical insurance and who have a strong co-pay or no co-pay on prescriptions. By using an online prescription company, save on your local pharmacy's inflated prices, and cut down the middle man efficiently. Most internet items are delivered either free of charge or on "x" dollar orders so you can buy products for three months to receive the free shipment. You save time and gas money right at your door.

3. I just read that 65 % of Americans had no dental coverage of any sort. I don't know if it's because of the present economy, the increasing cost of health insurance, or the common belief that dental plans are expensive. In any event, preventive maintenance is essential for your teeth. Take it from someone who needs thousands of dollars of painful work after years of neglect. Biannual cleaning and preventive treatment are the keys to saving dental care money. Some basic dental plans are surprisingly cost-effective and can help you get the basic prevention care you need.

4. There are several (natural) holistic home remedies for common web distress. I know that many of you may see this as an extent, but a few of them have been seen since late in various morning shows, newspapers, and other media sources. These are obviously of less serious, more

irritating kinds of conditions, such as eczema, acne, foot of athletes, etc. However, you can save money from what I saw here because it costs around as much as your average co-pay to see the doctor, and there are no drugs or creams to buy later. The best part of it is that most of all, I saw came with a money-back guarantee of 30-60 days. There's no risk in trying them, therefore.

In summary: it's not easy to be in the middle class. With poverty always out of reach on your head and wealth, you have to be diligent and practical in order to survive. Comparing health insurance, ordering prescription medicines online, searching for holistic medicinal products, and preventative maintenance through a cheap dental plan is just a couple of ways to save money.

We will just step back and look at what we really need to do now. This means for most of us to give up the little luxuries we have missed, so we will save every cent.

You need to change your life in order to lose weight and keep it away. It is more than picking different foods and adding more things to your day to change your lifestyle. It also involves changing the way you eat and work, which means changing your thinking, feeling, and doing.

Research has shown that a number of tools and tips help you improve effectively. Follow these changes tips:

Motivate yourself: Nobody can convince you to lose weight. In fact, increased pressure from people near you can only make things worse. Likewise, it is unusual to try to shed weight to impress anyone else. Create your own diet and fitness changes.

Make lifestyle changes a priority: Make sure you had already resolved other pressing challenges in your life as you plan to launch new lifestyle changes related to weight. It takes a lot of energy to change habits as well as you want to be sure that you concentrate on the subject at hand.

Plan: Develop a strategy that will change habits and attitudes gradually, which could have undermined the past efforts to lose weight. Select a certain start date. Think about how much you're going to run and how long. Determine a practical meal schedule with lots of meat, fruit, and vegetables. Write down everything about the plan as follows: When and where will you take your schedule, how will your plan fit, what possible roadblocks, and how might you deal with them.

Surround oneself with good examples: it helps surround you with good examples while setting your goals. Healthy lifestyle and nutritious eating magazines contain numerous real-life stories, safe and simple recipes, workout advice, and wellness facts.

Avoid food triggers: Avoid the desire to eat with something positive, like a friend. Say "NO" to fatty foods and large servings. Eat if you're hungry, not when it is time to eat the clock. Focus on eating when you eat. Serve your meal on smaller dishes to make it look like more food. Shop meals out of reach in general and should not keep fast-food around.

Keep a record: test yourself to lose weight. Hold a record: Keep a daily food and activity diary so you can strengthen good habits and discover and improve behaviors. Notice that performance is not only determined by the physical loss of weight. Check other important parameters of health, including blood pressure, cholesterol levels, and fitness overall.

Concentrate on the positive: Focus on what you can eat instead of focusing on what you cannot eat. Look at the new tastes and activities that your health will improve.

Don't give up: so much conspires in our culture to keep you overweight. You 're going to have reversed. Don't expect perfection right away. But don't give up, don't give up. Use recurrences to get on track. Motivate yourself when you reach your goals with healthy rewards.

Dealing with obesity can mean looking at how you live and making some difficult changes. If you are overweight or obese, you have to take a positive approach before you can throw out the unwanted pounds. You can and will lose weight safely, rapidly, and efficiently with knowledge, the right attitude, a good plan, and MRT complex.

www.ingramcontent.com/pod-product-compliance
Lightning Source LLC
Chambersburg PA
CBHW070811240726
48654CB00007B/306